Intermittent Fasting for Women Over 50

A New Healthy Lifestyle. How to Easily Lose 13lb in 45 Days or Less, Boost Your Immune System & Delay Aging. Easy Meal Plans and 7-Day Exercise Routines Included.

Lucy Solomon

This book is dedicated to my father, Solomon Kamau Gichuhi, who passed away in May 1997.
His devotion to God, determination to succeed and caring and courteous personality ultimately inspired me to write this book.
My love and thoughts are with you every day, Baba!

Contents

"If you don't do what's best for your body, you're the one who comes up on the short end."

— Julius Erving

Introduction

Few things are as difficult as trying to lose weight when you are over 50 years old. Your metabolism is much slower because you have lost a lot of your lean muscle mass. It doesn't help that your body seems to rebel against any activity that was easy when you were younger. The stubborn fat just won't budge. Fortunately, that doesn't have to be the case. With a few lifestyle changes, you can lose that fat and look forward to a healthy future. I will show you how in this book. But first, let me tell you a story.

It was the beginning of 2019. Laura was fed up. She was 52 years old and weighed 225 pounds. She hated her body. When she went outside to play with her four-year-old grandchild, she would have to stop to catch her breath. When they went to the park, they would be forced to sit down several times. Her second grandchild was just a few months old, and Laura was starting to worry that she would not be fit enough to play with her. She was also very aware of the risk of developing hypertension and diabetes, which run in her family. She knew that something had to give.

When Laura had her last child twenty years ago, she lost weight by running and changing her diet. Back then, she trained for half marathons, occasionally went to the gym, and watched what she ate. Laura had expected to be able to do the same when, in 2017, she tried to lose some weight. She tried running, but she soon realized that would not work. She resolved to watch her diet. That also did not work because she became obsessed with food. She was in that diet mindset for a few months and constantly policed what she ate.

When 2017 ended without much progress, Laura lost hope and returned to her old eating habits. By 2018, she had gained more weight and weighed 225 pounds. She didn't see a path forward for losing weight. Then, as if by divine intervention, in January 2019, she came across intermittent fasting. She was initially skeptical but thought there was no harm in trying. For her, the plan was simple. She would limit her eating to eight hours between 11 a.m. and 7 p.m. Five months of doing this while eating a balanced diet saw her lose 30 pounds. That was the time she accepted that it was legitimate. She added exercise into her plan, and within no time, she was within five pounds of what she weighed when she married at 23.

Laura's story could be your story too. Some women are cautious about dieting, having tried many diets and found them ineffective. Maybe you are like that. Perhaps, it seems like you are gaining weight uncontrollably even though you have not changed your eating habits, and you don't know what to do about it. Or perhaps, you have just reconciled with the aging process, are worried about your health and whether you will get to see your grandchildren grow up, and all you want is a plan that will get you healthy without breaking your back.

Perhaps you are going through menopause, and you want to do what it takes to remain healthy and young for your sake and the sake of your family. Maybe you tried a few diets but found that you didn't have the drive to stick with them. Intermittent fasting is the solution you have been looking for. This book is a detailed guide to intermittent fasting. You will learn the different intermittent fasting methods, or IF, as I will refer to it from here. We will explore all four methods to help you figure out which one will work best for you. Like Laura, you can lose weight quickly and live a healthier life through fasting. However, I go a little further with this book. Not only do I introduce you to IF, but I also have provided meal plans that you can use to eat healthily and exercises that you can do without risking injury to speed up the weight loss process. It is a one-stop shop for your weight loss journey.

I have lived through it all. I have seen the harsh realities of aging as a woman over 50. I have struggled to lose weight. I have tried diets that backfired on me. I have had nights when I could not sleep, worried about my health and the looming threat of hypertension. A few years ago, when I first encountered IF, I was just as cautious as you might be. I decided to put my research skills to learn about it. I read every book I could get my hands on, and then I jumped into the world of science. I pored over journal articles and research studies. I wanted to know what evidence there was supporting the legitimacy of IF.

Little by little, I was won over. I started IF myself. I experimented a bit with different meal plans and tried all the methods of IF, trying to get that sweet spot that would suit me best. Along the way, I discovered people who had fasted intermittently for years and were now living the kind of life I could only hope for. That inspired me to keep going. I read more about how fasting can reverse diabetes and hypertension. I found out what principles I could use to determine what to eat. I love to eat; I love food, and I love to cook. I didn't want to give any of that up. I tried to find a way that would support those loves.

Now, I am at a place in my journey where I am comfortable in my body. I have enjoyed the improved confidence IF brought me. I have seen my body transform, and each change has fueled my desire to keep living a healthy lifestyle. I am writing to help you make the same journey. My mother brought me up to pass along what I have learned, and that is, in part, what I hope to do with this book. I want to empower you to take charge of your health. With the information, meal plans, and exercises you find in this book, you can, as much as possible, guarantee that you not only lose weight but have a healthier life filled with energy and active days and a brighter future for yourself and your loved ones. If that sounds like what you are looking for, keep reading.

Chapter 1
All About Intermittent Fasting

There are many ways to lose weight, some involving diets, some focusing more on exercise, and others combining both. Of course, each option has its difficulties–some are more demanding than others. Intermittent fasting has become popular in recent years because it keeps things simple and helps you work toward your health goals. Generally, the eating pattern involves sustained and short-term fasts or periods of minimal to zero food consumption. It involves fasting for short periods, which helps you eat fewer calories and lose weight over time.

When someone says that they are trying to lose weight, they mean that they are trying to reduce body fat percentage. In an ideal dieting pattern, you don't lose muscle mass or much water weight. Research shows that IF is as close to ideal as it gets. It can help you lose fat while maintaining muscle mass more effectively than other low-calorie diets. In one review study, IF enabled people to reduce four to seven percent of their waist circumference in six months. They also lost excess belly fat, which is often harmful.

These findings line up with another recent study that considered evidence from people who had been fasting intermittently. Researchers found that test subjects who fasted intermittently lost 8.4lb more fat than those following a diet that required eating less than 800 calories per day. Imagine that! For women over 50, IF could help with weight loss and lower the chances of developing age-related illnesses. Research by the Baylor College of Medicine found that IF can lower blood pressure. Baylor College researchers were trying to understand hypertension and its relation to gut microbiota. They first established that hypertension does not develop because of gut dysbiosis (disruption of gut microbiota). Instead, it causes it. Then they set out to answer two questions – can you manipulate the microbiota to prevent or heal hypertension, and how do gut microbes influence blood pressure? Without going into unnecessary details about the research, the results showed that fasting lowers blood pressure by altering and reshaping gut microbiota.

However, for women over 50, the concern is not just about losing weight. They also want to improve their health, and many factors make it tougher to do so after 50 years. For starters, women over 50 suffer from achy joints and sleep issues. They often have a reduced muscle mass and lower metabolism. For them, however difficult, losing weight is essential to reduce the risk of health issues like cancer, heart attacks, and diabetes. Under these circumstances, IF can be seen as a fountain of youth and health.

Time-restricted patterns of eating have been found to prevent hypertension. A study in 2016 looked into combining resistance training and IF and found that participants could lose weight without impairing muscle strength or losing muscle. Another study compared different IF methods to other low-calorie diets and found that participants on IF ate 35% fewer calories than their counterparts without the stress of constant food obsession observed with calorie-counting diets. They also lost 7.7 pounds more within the first four weeks.

I could go on highlighting the research because there is no shortage of facts and data in support of IF. Researchers have even looked into the sustainability of IF and found that it can influence hormone levels in a positive and life-sustaining way. It helps increase HGH (human growth hormone) levels which are believed to burn fat faster. There is no need to keep beating the drum. The simple fact is that IF not only makes it easier to lose weight and keep it off, it also reduces the risks of developing health complications like hypertension and makes it easier to eat healthily. It is a dietary pattern that you can use for the rest of your life, and isn't that one of the key things to look for in a diet? This chapter will explore what IF is and how it works. This will set the foundation for the rest of this book.

What is intermittent fasting?

Most diets focus on what you eat, but IF is unique in focusing on when you eat. It is a dietary pattern that dictates the time you eat. It involves fasting for a certain period of your day or eating only one meal every day for several days every week. Scientific evidence points to the fact that it assists in weight loss. One researcher, Mark Mattson, who has been looking into different aspects of IF for over twenty-five years, says that our bodies evolved to go for hours or days without food. Before we learned to farm during prehistoric times, we were hunters and gatherers. Therefore, we knew how to survive without needing to eat for long periods. Our bodies developed this way because it took a lot of energy and time to hunt game or gather berries and nuts.

It was easier for people to sustain a healthy weight back then. There were no TV shows or computers. More people lived, played, and worked outside, which meant they exercised more. Today, we stay awake for long periods playing games, chatting online, or dealing with the ever-present needs of our digitally-oriented "always-on" world. We spend most of our days and nights seated and snacking. As a result, we have a higher risk of lifestyle illnesses like obesity and diabetes. IF is about going back to more beneficial patterns of eating. It combines periods of eating and fasting without specifying what you should eat.

IF is about returning to eating practices that served us better as human beings and embracing an approach that has existed throughout human evolution – fasting. It can be argued that fasting is more natural than eating three meals or more every day. No wonder many religions recommend fasting as a spiritual discipline. There are different forms of intermittent fasting, and we will explore them in Chapter Two, but what happens in the body is the same, regardless of the method you practice. Your body moves through a fed-fast cycle that involves different changes in your hormone and metabolism levels. The fed-fast cycle causes metabolic changes that help with weight loss and provides other health benefits. It has the following stages:

- **Fed state**

The fed state is the period that occurs within the first three hours after eating when your body is digesting and absorbing nutrients from food. During the fed state, your blood sugar level increases, and your body secrets higher insulin amounts. Insulin is the hormone that transports sugar into the cells from the blood. The amount of insulin your body releases depends on what you eat, how many carbs are consumed, and how sensitive your body is to insulin. Excess sugar gets stored in the muscles and liver as glycogen. Glycogen can be re-converted to sugar to provide your body with energy. In addition, other hormones like ghrelin and leptin are released during the fed state. Ghrelin is a hunger-stimulating hormone. It decreases during this stage. Leptin is appetite-suppressing, and it increases in the fed state. Remember that the fed-fast cycle will reset to this first state as soon as you eat.

- **Early fasting state**

Approximately four hours after eating, your body enters the early fasting state, which lasts until eighteen hours after your meal. Your insulin and blood sugar levels decline during the early fasting state, and your body starts producing glucose from glycogen for energy. When this stage is nearly at an end, your body runs out of glycogen in the liver and starts looking for an alternate energy source. It breaks down other fat cells into tiny molecules to supply its energy needs. It also converts amino acids into energy.

- **Fasting state**

You enter the fasting state eighteen hours to two days after starting fasting. At this point, there is no glycogen in the liver, and your body relies on protein and fat energy stores. As a result, it produces ketone bodies – the compound produced when fat is converted to fuel. Your body enters a metabolic state called ketosis, which uses fat as the primary energy source. Bear in mind that you do not enter ketosis immediately after you start fasting. The composition and size of your last meal affect how soon you enter ketosis.

During ketosis, you may experience decreased appetite, bad breath, fatigue, weight loss, and increased levels of ketone bodies in the urine, breath, and blood. Other diets like the ketogenic diet are about reaching ketosis, but IF involves shorter fasting windows and does not always induce this state. Remember that ketosis is not the same as ketoacidosis. Ketoacidosis is dangerous and means that your blood is too acidic. It results from illness and requires treatment.

- **Starvation/long-term fasting state**

When you have been fasting for an extended period, typically about forty-eight hours after a meal, your body enters a starvation state. Your insulin levels continually decrease during this state while BHB (beta-hydroxybutyrate – a ketone body) levels steadily increase. Your kidneys continue generating sugar through gluconeogenesis to fuel your brain. Your body also reduces the breakdown of essential amino acids to conserve muscle tissue. As a general rule of thumb, long fasts lasting more than two days are not recommended unless under medical supervision.

IF is currently very popular in the fitness and health community for its numerous benefits and other reasons.

Some people love its connection to modes of living many years before their time – to prehistoric times. Others love that IF gives them a structure around which they can eat healthily. Still, others love it for the discipline it introduces into their lives. Fortunately, IF is not so complicated that it needs extreme willpower like other diets; it does not exclude any food groups. You only need a clock to get started. That is part of its appeal. Finally, people love IF because it inevitably moves you toward healthy eating. When you have been fasting for three months and can see results of living the kind of life you want, you feel motivated to make positive eating and lifestyle changes, and isn't that like having the icing on the proverbial cake?

How does IF work?

Several things happen in your body on a molecular and cellular level when you fast. The types of changes in your body during IF can be categorized into two: metabolic and cellular changes. For example, your body adjusts its hormone levels to make stored body fat more accessible, and your cells begin to repair themselves. Hormones are the chemical messengers your body uses to carry out complex processes like metabolism and growth. They also manage your weight by modifying your appetite and the amount of fat you burn or store. According to studies, IF helps to balance fat-burning hormones.

When you fast, your body's HGH (human growth hormone) levels rise to five times their typical levels. This helps in fat loss and muscle building. According to recent studies, increases in HGH levels help in fat burning and muscle preservation. Secondly, fasting enhances your insulin sensitivity and lowers your blood insulin levels. When insulin levels are lower, your body fat is more accessible. Insulin, it turns out, is involved in fat metabolism, as it tells the body when to break down fat and when not to. As a result, having high insulin levels makes losing weight more difficult. Insulin levels are reduced by 20 to 31 percent with IF.

Finally, fasting helps to restart cellular healing. Your body undergoes autophagy after a few hours of fasting. Autophagy is a process by which your cells consume and eliminate old and defective proteins that have accumulated inside them. Fasting also changes gene expression. It affects the genes linked to illness resistance and longevity, allowing you to live longer. The many health benefits of intermittent fasting are due to these hormonal, cell function, and gene expression changes.

Fasting boosts your metabolism, making it a more effective weight-loss strategy than traditional calorie restriction. According to research, short-term fasting raises your metabolic rate. Long-term fasting may force your body to react by slowing down its metabolic rate to conserve energy but short-term fasting, as practiced in IF, is beneficial to your health. In one study, researchers looked at the metabolic changes of eleven healthy males while fasting. Their metabolism increased by 14 percent after three days of fasting. How impressive is that? The metabolic increase is usually caused by the rise in the hormone norepinephrine, which is involved in fat burning. It's also true that while you fast, you eat fewer times and less often. As a result, you take in fewer calories and burn more. That caloric deficit, of course, results in weight loss.

The pros of intermittent fasting

Let us now do a deep dive into some of the things you stand to gain from trying out and sticking to IF.

1. It helps with weight and visceral fat loss.

Most people who try IF do it hoping to lose weight, and it works every time. In general, when fasting intermittently, you eat fewer meals, so you will end up in a caloric deficit unless you overcompensate by overeating between fasts. Besides, as I have already demonstrated, IF enhances hormone function and facilitates weight loss. Simply put, IF helps you by working on both sides of the caloric equation. On the one hand, fasting increases your metabolic rate and enables you to burn more calories. On the other hand, you eat less. IF has been shown to cause a 3 to 8 percent weight loss when you start.

2. It reduces the risk of developing diabetes.

The recent decades have seen an increase in type 2 diabetes. The illness is characterized by high blood sugar levels due to insulin resistance. So anything that will lower your insulin resistance protects you against diabetes type 2. Fasting, in particular, does that. IF has been found to reduce blood sugar by between 3 and 6 percent in less than three months for people with prediabetes. It lowers insulin levels by between 20 and 31 percent.

3. It reduces oxidative stress.

Oxidative stress refers to the imbalance between antioxidants and free radicals in your body. As you age, you tend to be more affected by oxidative stress. The extra free radicals react with other molecules like DNA and proteins, leading to cell damage. Research has linked IF with increased resistance to oxidative stress. It also helps fight inflammation, a common problem associated with oxidative stress.

4. It helps to make your heart healthier.

Heart disease is one of the biggest killers in the world today. There are known risk factors associated with increased risk of heart diseases, such as obesity and an unhealthy diet. IF improves many of those risk factors, including blood pressure, inflammatory markers, blood sugar levels, and obesity, thus improving your heart's health.

5. It helps to repair your cells.

As mentioned earlier, when you fast, your body cells begin a cellular repair process – autophagy. Autophagy involves the breakdown and removal of dysfunctional proteins inside the cell. Increased autophagy protects you against many diseases, including cancer.

6. Helps in the prevention of cancer.

The hallmark of cancer is uncontrolled cell growth. Because it initiates autophagy, fasting helps in the prevention of cancer. There is also evidence that fasting reduces the side effects of chemotherapy for cancer patients undergoing treatment.

7. It may benefit the brain.

In most cases, whatever is good for the body, is good for the brain. Since IF improves many metabolic features, it benefits brain health. Studies show that IF could also increase new nerve cell growth, which helps brain function. Besides, fasting increases the levels of BDNF (Brain-derived neurotrophic factor), whose deficiency is linked with depression and other brain-related issues.

8. It may help to reduce Alzheimer's.

Alzheimer's is the most common neurodegenerative disease globally and has no cure, so preventing it is a good idea. Animal studies have linked fasting with the delay of early-onset Alzheimer's. Fasting has been found to reduce its severity. Different medical professionals typically use fasting as a lifestyle intervention to improve the symptoms of the disease.

9. Fasting helps you live longer.

In a world where a lot of research funding is going into finding ways to extend life, it is surprising that not many people think about natural ways to achieve longer life, like fasting. IF can extend your lifespan — it does this the same way as continuous calorie restriction. Daily fasting also improves your overall health by delaying the onset of conditions that threaten life or lower its quality. So yes, IF is just as good, if not better, than your anti-aging facial cream.

The cons of intermittent fasting

Like with most other things, there are arguments against IF, but after reading about them, you will find that the pros outweigh the cons.

1. It could cause you to overeat.

One study noted how many people gave up IF – there was a 38 percent dropout rate. It became clear that no one could sustain the diet for long if they got into it under duress or on impulse. Most of them ended up overeating, which affected their results, so they dropped out. It is human nature to want a reward after working hard, in this case, fasting. The danger is always to overindulge on non-fasting days. Some researchers say there is even a strong biological push to overeat after fasting because your hormones go into overdrive. It doesn't help that meal frequency and size are unrestricted in the feasting stage of IF. Consumers get to eat what they want during that period when they want it. The results? Overeating.

2. It may reduce your physical activity.

You may decrease your physical activity significantly when fasting. Most types of IF do not have a physical activity recommendation, so your lifestyle may become more sedentary unless you are intentional enough to include it.

3. It could leave you tired.

If we are honest, we can accept that most social interactions occur over food and drinks. Therefore, you will need a lot of willpower not to indulge while fasting. In some cases, fasting will call you to find alternatives so that you can have a social life and maintain your fast. This may be hard, but it is doable. Even so, fasting can make you tired. Despite the logistics that support it, you will have lower energy levels when fasting, and you may not feel the urge to move around as much as you did before.

4. It could cause an eating disorder.

People whose lifestyle is already active, or those on the leaner side, need to consult a doctor before fasting. IF could lead to hormonal imbalances, which could cause increased stress and insomnia, among other problems. Besides, without a careful watch over bodily functions and your emotional state during fasting, it could trigger eating disorders like anorexia. As a rule of thumb, avoid fasting if you have high caloric needs – that is, if you are pregnant, breastfeeding, or underweight. Fasting causes your blood sugar to drop to very low levels. You should also be careful if you have risk factors for developing an eating disorder. One of the factors is having a family member dealing with perfectionism, mood instability, impulsivity, and an eating disorder like bulimia.

The side effects of IF

Studies into the benefits of IF have also found that participants experience specific side effects during the fasting stage. It is not uncommon for them to feel tired, moody, constipated, or experience heartburn. Bear in mind that you may never experience all of them at once. Here are the most common side effects.

- **Hunger** – Hunger may become more severe when those around you eat regular snacks or meals.
- **Cravings** – Any restrictive diet will change how you interact with food. Some people may focus too much on food when fasting, which could cause orthorexia. But even if it doesn't get to that, most people experience cravings, so you may long for certain foods when you are in the fasting window.
- **Headaches** – They commonly occur during the early days of fasting. Fasting headaches are located in the frontal brain region and are often associated with low blood sugar. In 2020, the research studied eighteen people on IF and most reported mild headaches.
- **Lightheadedness** – It's the feeling that you might faint. Your body feels heavy, and your brain feels deprived of blood. Low blood sugar associated with IF is often responsible for lightheadedness.
- **Digestive issues** — Any diet could cause stomach upsets if you are not getting enough fiber, fluid, vitamins, or protein. Therefore, it is essential to eat a healthy diet during the eating

period and keep hydrating all day while fasting to avoid digestive issues.

- **Mood changes** – Moodiness is very common at the beginning of IF. Some people get an energy boost, but others experience a dip in their motivation as their bodies adjust to fasting. Feeling obligated to stick with IF could also affect your mood. Extreme mood changes may signify that you need a different fasting schedule for your body and mind.

- **Irritability** – Some people become very irritable when fasting due to low blood sugar. Irritability is often coupled with poor concentration. Funnily enough, according to research, while you may be irritable, you are also likely to experience a higher sense of pride and achievement at the end of the fasting period.

- **Fatigue** – Have you ever found yourself constantly yawning mid-morning, only to remember that you did not eat breakfast? Most people practicing IF choose to skip breakfast, which leaves them wading through the day feeling extremely tired. Fatigue may also kick in if you are not eating the right foods to stay healthy and strong.

- **Low energy** – During fasting, your body is running on less energy than usual, which means you may experience low energy levels as you go about your day, especially in the first days of attempting IF.

- **Bad breath** –Bad breath is a side effect that can occur during fasting. This is caused by a lack of salivary flow and the rise of acetone in the breath. After breaking your fast, your salivary glands begin stimulating again, and your bad breath disappears. Bad breath may also be caused by your body going into ketosis. Ketone bodies used to fuel the body during ketosis have a metallic smell that manifests as bad breath.

- **Sleep disturbances** – Some people experience improved sleep patterns after starting IF because it helps them stop their late-night snacking habits. Others report sleep disturbances. IF causes a decrease in REM (rapid-eye movement) sleep, which means a more disturbed sleeping pattern.

- **Dehydration** – You get 20 percent of your daily fluid requirements from food. So, even if you usually drink water but are not eating, you risk dehydration during fasting. That is why it is essential to hydrate constantly. Besides, early in the fast, when your body burns glycogen, it releases water into your blood, but when those stores are depleted, you need extra hydration because no more water is removed.

- **Malnutrition** – IF can lead to unhealthy eating habits if not done correctly. Be careful not to mess up your diet during the non-fasting hours, as you could not get enough nutrients from your food.

Now you know what IF is. We have explored what it entails and how it affects your body in the different fasting stages. We have even considered the pros and cons of IF and its side effects. It is time to learn more about the types or forms of intermittent fasting that can be incorporated into your days.

Chapter 2
The Types of Intermittent Fasting

This chapter will detail the forms of intermittent fasting and their benefits, but before I dig into that, let me tell you Sophia's story. Sophia started her IF journey at 230 pounds, and in one year, she had lost 100 pounds with IF and mild exercise. She first learned about it by chance when she stumbled upon a group on Facebook where women used an app to track their progress. She noticed that some of her friends were in the group, so her curiosity was piqued. She thought that these women had just chosen not to eat. How do you go without breakfast and lunch, she wondered to herself.

Still, more out of curiosity than any innate desire to change her lifestyle, Sophia stayed in the group and started following what the other women were doing. She noticed that some women reported feeling better after fasting. One woman even said that IF helped reverse her diabetes. To Sophia, this sounded too good to be true. She was a bit apprehensive, but since her friends were doing it, she resolved that she would continue for one month, only to see if their claims had merit.

Soon enough, Sophia learned that there are many IF options. She tried the six hours of eating and eighteen hours of fasting option and found it very challenging. She fell off the wagon a few times, but it started feeling normal to her after two weeks. She realized that there were times she would be hungrier than at other times. She started drinking more water and tea. It helped the waves of hunger to pass. When hunger seemed all-consuming, she would choose to focus on something else, provided it was not during her eating window. Skipping breakfast was not a problem, and sometimes, she would push herself to start eating at 2 p.m. and finish at 6 p.m.

After one month, Sophia had become familiar with how IF worked. She started adding long fasts to her plan. She would fast for 48 hours straight every week for two months. Within three months of starting, she had lost 35 pounds and was eating only within a three-hour window a day. It was now no longer about following her friends. It had become personal. She was starting to own her journey and body and she loved it. So, Sophia decided that she needed another challenge. She would eat only one meal every day. She could always revert to her regular schedule if it didn't work. The meal would be dinner, and she would share it with her family. She decided that she would not restrict her food.

Sophia also decided to allow herself a longer eating window during the holidays to celebrate with her loved ones. She wanted to still be able to enjoy herself. By this time, she had lost 50 pounds, but her body was not the only thing that had changed. She was also becoming more confident. She learned how to use social media and started posting her journey and what she was learning on Instagram. Nothing had prepared her for how much she would enjoy using social media and how valuable her accounts would be to women her age. Sophia was 45 years old at this point. She was indeed becoming a better wife, mother, and friend.

While experimenting with one meal daily, Sophia would start with chips, guac, and nuts. Somedays, she would eat rice, beans, cabbage, or a salad. On other days she would eat cheese and eggs. Her idea was to have a satisfying meal and share it with her loved ones before she was done for the day. She ensured the meal was as healthy as possible, knowing she would not eat until the next day. It took a while for her body to get used to it, but it became a habit when she got into the rhythm. In one year, owing to her newfound confidence, Sophia had lost over 100 pounds and made changes to her life that she would never have imagined possible.

Sophia started IF by chance, but she was wise enough to take stock of her life and be willing to do something to help herself, even though it initially seemed strange. It took her a while before she accepted that her past lifestyle was unsustainable. When she started IF, she was bold enough and honest enough with herself to experiment with different methods; she didn't want to be so rigid that she would give up before trying. That is the point of learning the various types of IF. When you understand the different options, you can see what works best for you, and you can tweak your fasting to make it more likely that you will stick with it until you reach your desired goals.

Bear in mind that proper nutrition is key during IF. Even though these types are similar, there is no one-size-fits-all when it comes to weight loss. You have to figure out which method to incorporate into your life and how it will affect things like social events and staying active. With that said, let's consider the five main methods of IF:

Time-Restricted Fasting

Time-restricted fasting is a form of fasting that limits the time of the day for eating. There are two main types of time-restricted fasting – the 16/8 method and the 14/10 method. This involves eating as much as you want during the eating window. Time-restricted fasting aims to align the fasting and eating cycles to your body's innate 24-hour circadian system. In humans, individual cells synchronize into circadian rhythms. There is evidence that cells have their own clocks. The clocks regulate gene expression and coordinate metabolism, so aligning your eating with them allows you to enjoy fasting benefits like weight loss and improved heart function without changing what or how much you eat.

During time-restricted fasting, you must set your eating and fasting windows well. Most people enjoy time-restricted IF because most of the fasting time can be scheduled to coincide with sleep, which makes it convenient. It is also the safest type for those just starting on IF. It can be repeated as often as you would like or even done twice a week, according to your preference. Remember that it may take a few days to figure out your ideal fasting and eating windows, especially if you are very active in the morning or wake up hungry.

- **Method #1: 16/8**

The 16/8 method is about limiting your food intake and intake of calorie-containing beverages to only eight hours every day. Then, you abstain from food for the remaining 16 hours but still drink water and zero-calorie drinks like tea or coffee. This method has become very popular because of its benefits, which we will discuss shortly. The 16/8 IF is easy to follow because it does not have many strict rules and still offers measurable results in a reasonable time. As a rule of thumb, eat high-fiber whole foods, stay hydrated throughout the day, and consult your doctor before starting if you have underlying health conditions.

Choosing a time window for this fasting method is relatively simple. Just audit your days and pick an eight-hour period for eating, then abstain from food afterward. The most popular time windows include:

- 7 a.m. to 3 p.m.
- 9 a.m. to 5 p.m.
- 12 p.m. to 8 p.m.
- 2 p.m. to 10 p.m.

The eating window can be any eight hours of your choice, but it may be wise to schedule it during the day so that you can fast overnight. Some people like to skip breakfast and begin their eating day at lunchtime. Others skip dinner because they need to eat breakfast to go about their day. Experiment with different timeframes and pick the one that works best with your schedule. You could set a time to alert you of the transitions at the start and end of your eating window.

The 16/8 method has many advantages, including its convenience. It can save you money and simplify your life as you spend less money and time cooking or preparing meals. It is also associated with health benefits such as:

- **Increased weight loss** – Reducing your eating window reduces your calorie intake throughout the day, leading to weight loss. Besides, research has shown this method yields higher weight loss in obese men than standard calorie restriction.

- **Improved control of your blood sugar levels** – This fasting method reduces your blood sugar and insulin levels, decreasing your risk of diabetes. It is also a promising intervention for people who have already been diagnosed with type 2 diabetes.

- **Extended longevity** – Research shows that people who started with the 16/8 method were able to stay on track with IF compared to those who began fasting with other forms. Over a couple of years, fasting helped improve their insulin sensitivity, creating behavioral changes that increased their lifespan.

- **Can prevent disease** – This method has been praised for helping prevent heart conditions, neurodegenerative diseases, and type 2 diabetes. The eight-hour eating window also helps lower blood pressure for adults with obesity. In addition, it protects memory and learning and slows down diseases that affect the brain.

The 16/8 method is sustainable, safe, and easy for people just beginning IF, especially if paired with a healthy lifestyle and nutritious diet.

- **Method #2: 14/10**

The 14/10 method is not as well-known as the 16/8 one, but it is as simple to follow, if not simpler. It is an eating pattern where you eat for ten hours a day and fast for the next fourteen hours. For example, if you get up early, you can set your ten-hour window to start at 7 a.m. and then eat your last meal for the day at 5 p.m. You can eat as you usually do during the eating window, but you must consume zero calories during the fast. Like with the 16/8 method, if you complement this method with a well-balanced and healthy diet, you will find it easy to lose weight and pivot to a healthier and more sustainable lifestyle. A study in 2019 found that fasting for more than ten hours in a day significantly benefits your blood pressure, weight, and metabolic health. Be sure to ease into it, though, if you have never fasted before.

Like with the 16/8 method, there are popular time windows for the 14/10 method, including:

- 7 a.m. to 5 p.m.
- 8 a.m. to 6 p.m.
- 9 a.m. to 7 p.m.

The general rule is to find the time window that will be easy for you to adapt to and follow. For example, the 7 a.m.to 5 p.m. window may work best if you wake up early. Remember that these windows are not written in stone. Keep the principle and adjust the time frame to suit your needs. The 14/10 has its advantages which include:

- **Reducing high blood pressure** – Studies show that eating for ten hours and fasting for the rest of the day increases cardiovascular health and lowers blood pressure, decreasing the risk of severe health conditions like obesity.

- **Lowering cholesterol levels** – Most studies on IF have focused on the 16/8 and 5/2, but some evidence shows that 14/10 fasting effectively improves your cardiometabolic health. It reduces your calorie intake and improves metabolic markers like insulin sensitivity. The body enters ketosis, and you start burning fat, causing a decrease in your cholesterol levels.

- **It is an easy starting place** – The 14/10 method is an excellent variant to try if you are having trouble with the 16/8 method. Some experts recommend starting with the 14/10 and then working up to other methods once your body is accustomed to missing some meals. For example, sleeping for an adult's recommended eight hours a day leaves you only six hours to fast. Besides, a ten-hour window for eating is enough to ease you into IF while still being practical for weight loss.

The Twice-a-Week Method

- **Method #3: 5/2**

The 5/2 IF method can be a very effective weight-loss tool if you eat right because the pattern generally helps you eat fewer calories. It is a fasting protocol whereby you reduce your food intake for two days every week. The method was popularized in 2013 by British TV journalist and former doctor Michael Mosley. His bestselling book outlined the method and launched it into the public psyche. Health and wellness enthusiasts have picked it up, tried it out, reviewed it, and tweaked it to suit their goals. Research shows that, like the 16/8 and the 14/20 methods, this IF method has many health benefits.

In 2021, the method, otherwise known as the 'fast diet,' was ranked among the best diets by *US News and World Report*. It is well-known for restricting people's overall caloric intake. However, some people have trouble getting used to it because, for the diet to work, they cannot compensate for the fasting days by overindulging on non-fasting days. Further research into the 5/2 method has shown that people lost 3-8 percent of their weight in six months. They also lost harmful body fat and retained their muscle mass.

The 5/2 method does have some calorie restrictions, though. Women must eat a maximum of 500 calories a day on fasting days, while men can eat up to 600 calories. On non-fasting days, you eat as you usually would, i.e., the number of calories your body needs for its daily functions (TDEE – total daily energy expenditure). You are also encouraged to eat a wide range of foods. However, for the 5/2 diet to work, you need simplicity. Do not complicate your meal plans or insist on measuring portions or counting calories. Instead, focus on the number of carbs you eat and the amount of protein in certain foods. You could even gain weight if you overeat high-sugar, high-calorie, or overly processed foods on eating days.

During your fasting days, experiment to find the best times to eat for your body and brain. Some people work best on a small breakfast, while others prefer to wait as long as they can bear it. The aim is to eat only 25 percent of your regular intake. Since your food intake is limited on fasting days, try to spread those calories as much as possible. For example, you can have 200 calories for breakfast, 100 for lunch, and 200 for dinner. If you prefer two meals a day, eat 250 calories at one meal and 250 calories at another. These are the two common meal patterns – light breakfast, lunch, and dinner or only lunch and dinner.

It is not simple to shift from regular eating to consuming only 500 calories daily on two days, so it is wise to ease into it. Slowly reduce your calorie consumption until you get to the desired amounts. For example, you can reduce your intake to 1500 calories from 2000 on the fasting days during the first week. Then, keep doing it until you get to 500 calories. Like other IF methods, there is no rule concerning what you eat, but focusing on high-protein, high-fiber foods that leave you feeling fuller for longer without increasing your caloric intake is wise.

You can expect overwhelming hunger during the first few days after starting the 5/2 method. It is also customary to feel slower or weaker than usual. However, the hunger fades fast if you keep busy, and after the first few fasts, it becomes easier. It is entirely up to you which days you choose to fast, but here is a sample schedule you could follow:

- Monday – Normal
- Tuesday – Fast
- Wednesday – Normal
- Thursday – Normal
- Friday – Fast
- Saturday – Normal
- Sunday – Normal

The 5/2 method has many benefits, including:

- **You can eat whatever you like** – No foods are forbidden; only the number of calories is limited during fasting. This method is straightforward and still schedules time to socialize with others so that you never feel deprived while fasting.

- **You can choose when to fast** – On the 5/2 diet, you are free to choose which days will be good for you to fast based on your schedule. You can plan your fasting days around social events and family gatherings.

- **Improves cardiovascular health** – A study by the American Journal of Clinical Nutrition found the plan excellent for people wanting to improve their cardiovascular health. In ten weeks, participants were already doing better than when they started fasting.

- **Improves metabolic health** – The 5/2 method aligns with the federal guidelines for a healthy and balanced diet on non-fasting days. On those days, eat nutrient-dense foods, including dairy products, grains, vegetables, and fruit, as per the USDA recommendations. On fasting days, your body enters ketosis and autophagy so that you return from fasting with a healthier metabolism.

Alternate-Day Fasting (ADF)

- **Method #4: ADF**

ADF is a version of intermittent fasting where you eat on one day and fast the following day. There are different modifications of the ADF method, but all of them involve eating every other day. Some versions allow you to eat a few calories during fasting, while others require that you take zero calories. ADF has health benefits like improving the biomarkers for heart health, aging, and metabolic well-being, which we will discuss in detail. It is generally safe for most people but is not advisable for pregnant or nursing women and children. If you have eating disorders or underlying health conditions, consult with your doctor before trying ADF.

Here is a sample of what ADF could look like:

- Monday – Normal
- Tuesday – Fast
- Wednesday – Normal
- Thursday – Fast
- Friday – Normal
- Saturday – Fast
- Sunday – Normal

Remember that the days will be different in the second week. For example, Monday would be a fast day in week

2, Tuesday would be a normal eating day, and so on. The alternation goes on for as long as you maintain ADF. You can modify the fasting plan to eat some calories on the fasting days, especially when you are just beginning, so it is not too challenging. Your calorie intake should be between 25 and 40 percent of your energy needs. This is anywhere between 400 and 700 calories per fasting day. If you are unsure about your daily energy needs, use the USDA guidelines or consult with a registered dietitian. Whether you modify your fasting plan or not, do not overindulge on the eating days to make up for all the calories you skipped during your fast. The point of the ADF is to lower your calorie intake.

To make it easier on yourself, on the fasting days, get your calories from foods high in water, fiber, and protein. They will fill you up, keep you hydrated, ward off hunger and distract you from your fasting. If you feel adventurous enough, you can also combine fasting with a high-fat, low-carb, or low-fat diet as you see fit. Either way, ADF has the following benefits:

- **Manages type 2 diabetes** – 90 percent of the 34 million Americans have type 2 diabetes. In addition, more than 30 percent of all American adults are prediabetic. ADF can help you fight against type 2 diabetes in two main ways. First, it helps you lose weight which can reverse diabetes symptoms and manage the risk factors. Secondly, fasting lowers your insulin levels, and ADF is best-suited for this because you fast for longer periods.

- **Improves heart health** – ADF is an excellent option for cardiac wellness. It helps you maintain a healthy weight which positively impacts your heart health. It does this by managing heart health biomarkers like blood pressure and cholesterol.

- **It stimulates autophagy** – Autophagy is a natural process whereby your body breaks down old cells and recycles them. It helps in disease prevention and managing chronic health conditions. It is also closely tied to the aging process. ADF boosts autophagy, leading to slower aging, increasing longevity, and fewer chances of developing tumors.

The 24-Hour Fasting

- **Method #5: Eat-Stop-Eat**

The eat-stop-eat method involves a complete fast for 24 hours at a time. You only do it once or twice a week. Some people fast from breakfast to breakfast while others prefer lunch to lunch. You typically fast for 24 hours before returning to your regular diet on your non-fasting days. This version of intermittent fasting can be extreme, especially for beginners, and could leave you feeling tired, irritable, and with low energy. After researching the effects of fasting on metabolic health, Brad Pilon developed the plan and wrote his book 'Eat Stop Eat.'

According to Pilon, while the method has other benefits, it is primarily about reevaluating what you have come to believe about meal frequency and timing and how those relate to your health. The eat-stop-eat method differs from the 5/2 method in that you do not eat anything for the 24 hours of fasting. Therefore, you may only need to fast for one day a week, not necessarily two. During the non-fasting days, though, you need to eat responsibly and watch to see what pattern of meals works best for you.

Implementing the eat-stop-eat method is pretty simple – you choose one or two days a week during which you fast and then abstain from food for 24 hours. For the other days of the week, you eat freely. It may seem complicated, but you eat on each calendar day of the week. For example, if you fast between 9 a.m. on Wednesday and 9 a.m. on Thursday, you can have your meal on Wednesday before 9 a.m. and Thursday after 9 a.m. Remember that you have to stay properly hydrated when practicing the eat-stop-eat method. The method has benefits such as:

- **Encourages weight loss** – Mounting evidence shows that periodic and sustained fasting in the eat-stop-eat method supports weight loss in most people. It allows your metabolism to rest and boosts it. When used with a reduced caloric intake, this leads to weight loss.

- **Shifts your metabolic state** – Your body experiences some metabolic shifts during fasting. Typically, it breaks carbs into glucose for energy. However, during the eat-stop-eat method, after twelve hours of fasting, your body enters ketosis and starts using fat for energy instead. Prolonged fasting keeps you in ketosis for longer, making it superior to other dieting strategies.

- **Lowers your caloric intake** – This is probably the most obvious way the eat-stop-eat method is beneficial. It reduces your caloric intake—you lose one to two days' worth of calories per week.

Now that you understand the different types of IF, which one are you interested in trying? To further help you make that choice, we will consider what your body is going through in the next chapter. The idea is to understand what you are fighting against to be better equipped to master intermittent fasting.

Chapter 3
The Aging Process of Your Body

"Age fast, age slow – it's up to you."

— Kenneth H. Cooper, MD, MPH.

Aging is gradual. It is a continuous and natural process. It begins in early adulthood into middle age, with many of your bodily functions gradually declining. Generally speaking, people do not become elderly at a specific age. Traditional societies thought sixty-five was the beginning of old age, but that was based on history, not biology. For example, Germany became the first country to mandate sixty-five as the age for retirement. It continues to be the retirement age in many developed societies even though that tradition is changing and people are beginning to choose when to retire.

You can think of old age chronologically. However, chronological age is only about the passage of time and how many years you have been alive. Thinking of aging this way has limited meaning in some ways, but you are indeed more likely to develop health problems as you age chronologically. No wonder chronologic age plays a role in some financial and legal issues. You can also think of aging biologically. Biological age is about the changes happening in your body as you age. As it is, these changes affect some people earlier than they do others.

It is worth mentioning that most of the noticeable differences in apparent age between people of a similar chronological age result from habit, lifestyle, and the effects of diseases and are not so much the result of actual aging. Finally, you can think of aging psychologically. Psychological age is based on how you feel and act. For instance, an eighty-year-old who works, anticipates and plans the future is psychologically young.

Most of the time, as people age, they wonder whether what they are going through is normal or abnormal. Although we age differently, some changes result from internal processes – aging itself. These changes are sometimes unwelcome, but they are normal. They are universal and generally unavoidable. This chapter will break them down. Here you will see the general changes people experience, but remember that what makes for normal aging is not always clear at the end of the day. Some people develop disorders, while others do not.

It also turns out that you can do things to compensate for some of the changes that come with aging. For example, older adults are likelier to lose teeth than their younger selves. Regular dentist appointments, flossing and brushing your teeth daily, and being more mindful of what you eat, could reduce tooth loss. In that sense, even though losing teeth is typical of old age, it is avoidable. As you read through this chapter and learn what to expect as you age, be empowered by what you learn. Think about what you could do now to prevent what is avoidable.

As it turns out, there is such a thing as successful or healthy aging. Healthy aging is about postponing or reducing the undesired effects of aging. The goal is to maintain mental and physical health, avoid diseases and stay independent and active. As you will see as you keep reading, IF helps you age successfully. The idea is that the sooner you develop healthy eating habits, the better. That way, you have more control over what happens to you as you age.

So yes, age gives you wisdom, experience, and strength. It allows you to develop meaningful relationships and watch people around you grow. You start to discover the things that truly matter to you, enabling you to let go of some of society's imposed rules that may have governed many of your younger days. But, along with those positives comes physical changes. You have probably experienced some of those changes, but what more subtle changes can you look out for? Here are some of the changes your body may go through after 50:

Expected changes after 50

1. The production of collagen in your body slows down.

Collagen is a body protein that forms the primary component in connective tissues. It gives your skin its structure and contributes to muscle and bone strength. Collagen is like a glue that keeps your muscles, bones, connective tissues, and skin together. It makes up about 75 percent of your skin's dry weight and contributes 30 percent of your body's total mass of proteins. There are over twenty-five types of collagen in your body, each serving a unique role. Type I collagen, for example, is responsible for providing skin, tooth, and bone structure.

Your body produces less collagen as you age, which explains why your skin loses some elasticity and firmness. Some research shows that collagen production starts to slow at 20 years of age at a rate of one percent per year. After 50, the production decreases even more. Science shows that lifestyle and environmental factors could worsen the situation.

2. Your skin becomes drier.

It is common to hear older women complain about dry and itchy skin, especially in winter. Sometimes the temperatures are to blame, but other times, it results from old age. As you age, your sweat glands and oil glands become less active. This makes it harder for your skin to stay moist. It also makes your skin more fragile. A recent survey involving over 3800 postmenopausal women found that 36 percent suffered from dry skin. Past 50, your body is experiencing hormonal shifts that change the performance of skin cells. This impairs its ability to repair and heal. Dry skin is also tied to a decreased production of estrogen. Drinking enough water may help your skin to bounce back and recover faster.

3. You hit menopause.

At around 50 years old, women begin experiencing menopause. This is because their ovaries produce less estrogen and progesterone and make more of the follicle-stimulating hormone. The extent to which these hormonal changes happen varies from person to person, but the effects of these changes include things like hot flashes, depression, mood swings, and insomnia. At menopause, the menstrual cycle stops entirely and permanently because your body has no more ovarian oocytes. Generally speaking, medical practitioners diagnose menopause after you miss your period for twelve consecutive months. Diagnosis often involves blood tests to measure hormone levels. Unfortunately, most women have to learn to manage the symptoms of menopause. Still, there are some treatments available to lower and control menopause symptoms until the body finds a new equilibrium.

4. Your bone density decreases.

As we age, we usually can't feel what is happening inside our bones, but throughout life, specialized cells constantly update the collagen framework supporting our body. It is like a never-ending road reconstruction project where old bone is broken down and replaced daily. This happens until you hit 25, so your bone density constantly increases. Between ages 25 and 50, your bone density stays stable, with equal amounts of bone formation and bone breakdown. However, after 50, bone breakdown gets faster, so bone loss accelerates. Lower bone density is a problem, particularly for older women; it is caused by dips in estrogen after age 50. Studies show that low bone density affects about forty-four million people in the US. According to reports from the National Osteoporosis Foundation, one out of every two women over 50 is likely to break a bone because of osteoporosis.

5. Your hair begins to thin.

Hair is made of protein strands with a lifespan of between two and seven years. On average, hair grows at about 0.5 inches per month and is affected by genetics, health, and diet. As you age, the life cycle of hair becomes shorter, and the more delicate hair falls out. It is replaced by new hair, which is also finer and manifests as thinning hair over time. Many factors increase the risk of hair thinning with age, including thyroid disorders, nutritional deficiencies, and hereditary traits. However, for women, menopause also plays a significant role.

During menopause, sex hormones that stimulate hair growth decrease, and your body has a slight testosterone dominance. Because of this, some hair follicles stop creating new hair. Over time, your hair fibers thin and drop out but never get replaced, hence, thinning. This whole process is also tied to pigment changes. The pigment cells stop producing as much pigment, so your hair begins to gray.

6. You experience trouble sleeping.

After 50, you may notice that you don't sleep as well as you used to. If this is you, do not panic. It does not necessarily translate to insomnia. The National Sleep Foundation says it is normal to experience sleep pattern changes after 50. You may have difficulty falling asleep, and when you do, you may wake up many times throughout the night. This is because, as you age, your body stops producing as much growth hormone as it did. This translates to less melatonin, resulting in fragmented sleep at night. It is also common to go to sleep earlier in the evening and wake up earlier than you used to.

7. You experience a slower heart rate.

After 50, you may have difficulty walking up the stairs or mowing the lawn as quickly as you used to. This is because age causes your heart rate to slow. The average heart muscle is the size of your clenched fist. It has different chambers that pump blood around the body. As you get older, your heart and blood vessels change. Fatty deposits in arterial walls over the years cause your heart to beat slower and increase your risk of heart disease. Besides that, your large arteries also become stiffer. This results in hypertension or high blood pressure.

8. Your bladder control decreases.

The kidneys filter blood and eliminate extra fluid and wastes from the body. They also control the chemical balance in the body. They are part of the urinary system, including the urethra, ureters, and bladder. As you age, your kidneys and bladder change, which affects their function. For example, your kidney tissue decreases with age, and you have fewer filtering units, which diminishes kidney function. Some blood vessels could also harden, slowing the operation of the kidneys.

At the same time, your bladder wall changes. It becomes stiffer, and your bladder becomes less stretchy, so the bladder cannot hold as much urine as it did when you were younger. Sometimes the urethra also becomes blocked, and the vagina falls out of position. These muscle and reproductive system changes can negatively affect bladder control and cause urinary incontinence.

9. Your bones shrink.

You may not realize it when it happens, but you do shrink with age. After age 40, the disks between your spine vertebrae start drying and thinning out, causing your spine to compress and you to shrink. Research shows that after 60, men may lose two inches of their height while women may lose an inch. Where the shrinking is significant, it could result from worn-out cartilage between the knee and hip joints. A decrease in muscle mass with age is also sometimes connected to a reduction in height. You have no cause to worry if you shrink a little, but if you notice yourself shrinking too fast, it may indicate a bigger problem. Losing two inches within a year is shrinking too fast — consult your doctor if this is the case.

10. Your night vision becomes worse.

So many conditions associated with old age could make it harder for you to see at night. It could be cataracts. As you age, cells inside your eyes grow and die. The buildup of dead cells causes cataracts that are not painful but slowly cloud your lens. Sometimes diminished night vision is the first sign of cataracts. They distort the light coming into your eyes, causing you to see halos around lights and blurring your vision. Other times, worsened night vision is a function of nutrient deficiencies like a lack of vitamin A or not having enough zinc in your body.

If you have been diagnosed with diabetes, years of high blood sugar could damage your eyes' nerves and blood vessels, causing blurred night vision. Prolonged sun exposure over the years may also contribute to diminished night vision, and so does diabetes. Whatever the cause, do not be surprised if you need reading glasses or brighter light to see at night after 50.

11. You struggle to deal with dry eyes.

As you get older, your tear glands produce fewer tears which could manifest as dry eyes. Women are particularly prone to dry eyes because of the hormonal changes wrought by menopause. In a functional eye, your eyes are lubricated by tears, so you suffer when your tear glands no longer produce as many tears. Other people make tears, but because they are poor-quality tears, they still experience dry eyes. Dry eyes feel like a burn or sting in the eyes. Sometimes they are situational, like when you are in an air-conditioned room, but other times you can see no apparent trigger. There are lifestyle changes and treatments that can help control dry eye symptoms.

12. You notice a decreased perception of color.

Even if you have never been color blind, you can lose your ability to tell between different hues after the age of 50. The American Optometric Association suggests that this is partly due to a discoloration in your eyes that interferes with your color perception. Your eyes become yellowish, and you feel like you are looking through a filter. Studies show that this color perception will continue to worsen with time. People over 70 often have trouble differentiating between blue and purple or yellow and green. Fortunately, this diminished color perception does not affect your life.

13. Your sweat smells different.

Body odor changes throughout life. Think of the distinct, fresh scent of a newborn baby or the smell of a teenage boy. It is the same with older adults. Many people describe that scent as musty. As you age, your hormone levels change, causing your sweat composition to change too.

Besides, age increases the production of a compound responsible for body odor known as 2-Nonenal. 2-Nonenal is one of the byproducts of the breakdown of Omega-7 unsaturated fatty acids. Other chemicals and compounds in your body can change with time too.

14. Your sense of taste and smell diminishes.

Smell and taste work together. You have more than 10,000 taste buds that sense savory, bitter, salt, sour, and sweet flavors. As you age, the number of these taste buds decreases and the remaining ones start shrinking. This causes their sensitivity to decline. Additionally, your mouth starts producing less saliva, which causes dry mouth and affects your sense of taste. As your sense of taste diminishes, so does your sense of smell. Research shows that after 50, you may lose nerve endings in your nose and produce less mucus. Mucus typically keeps odors in the nose long enough for you to smell them, so as it reduces, so does your sense of smell.

15. Your immune system gets weaker.

Your immune system protects your body from harmful or foreign substances such as viruses, bacteria, and toxins. It makes antibodies and cells that destroy toxic substances. As you age, your immune system grows weaker because of specific changes in the body. It responds more slowly to harmful substances, increasing your risk of catching the flu. Vaccines or flu shots do not work as well as previously. Some people develop an autoimmune disorder that causes the immune system to attack itself by mistake so that it damages healthy body tissues. The immune system's ability to find and correct cells declines, increasing the risk of cancer. It also means that your cells heal slower and have fewer immune cells.

16. Your metabolism changes.

Once you reach 30, your metabolism begins to decline. By the time you are 50, your metabolism has slowed down by about 15 percent, primarily due to lost muscle. It turns out that muscle burns more calories than fat when at rest. It may mean that you have lost muscle if you notice yourself feeling significantly weaker or tired after taking a walk. An AARP and Abbott survey surveyed 1500 people and found that 73 percent of participants understood that we lose muscle with age, but only 13 percent of them realized why it is crucial to maintain muscle mass as they aged. According to the survey, most respondents were worried about losing muscle and strength due to chronic disease after 50.

17. You experience unexpected weight gain.

It is not uncommon to gain weight unexpectedly after 50 even though you have not changed your eating and life-style habits. According to the CDC, women tend to gain a lot of belly fat after menopause. The International Menopause Society does not think menopause causes weight gain, but the hormonal changes happening during this time are to blame. Besides, as you age, your cells become more resistant to insulin. When you are insulin resistant, your cells do not readily absorb blood sugar from the bloodstream, which keeps your blood sugar levels high and increases the risk of developing diabetes. Insulin resistance causes weight gain around the belly area.

18. Your joints get weaker.

Typically, your bones are not in direct contact with a joint. Instead, they have cartilage lining them and serving as cushioning. Joints also have synovial membranes and a lubricating fluid inside them. As you grow older, your joint movements become stiffer and less flexible because of reduced lubricating fluid in the joints and thinning cartilage. Your ligaments also shorten, contributing to the loss of flexibility. You can mitigate against most of these changes by exercise. Moving the joint helps to keep the fluid moving.

As I mentioned earlier, these changes happen at different times for different people. The tendency is usually to imagine that there is nothing you can do about them and to age successfully. Yet, taking charge of your health is a significant step in the right direction, which is where IF comes in. Contrary to popular folklore, IF is not unhealthy. It is not about starving yourself. It is about being proactive regarding your health. In the next chapter, we will debunk some of the myths associated with intermittent fasting that may be fueling some of your fears surrounding IF.

Chapter 4
Debunking the Myths of Intermittent Fasting

Thanks to technology and the internet, people today have more access to data and information than ever before. Social networking sites are used to obtain information on all sorts of topics – you can learn about your son's job, your grandchild's school, or connect with a colleague from ten years ago. Everything you ever wanted to know is at your fingertips. Now, you don't need to spend hours in a library looking for the perfect book to learn about a subject you are interested in. Unfortunately, not only is it true that information is easily accessible and spreads rapidly on the internet – misinformation spreads just as fast.

Studies show that many Americans, for example, cannot tell what is real and what is fake news. Of course, this causes misunderstanding, confusion, and, often, polarization. As it turns out, there is a lot of misinformation or fake news regarding IF—which is doing its share of harm.

Imagine being in school, doing your research, and submitting your paper only to discover that your sources of information were unreliable. What does that do to you? You fail. Myths have a similar effect.

Myths can have adverse effects. For example, misleading stories about something as crucial as IF could result in you either fasting incorrectly or not fasting at all, and in both cases, you put your health at risk. Believing the myths may cause you to make harmful decisions about your health. Misinformation or fake news can make it harder for you to see the truth about IF. A study conducted by Pew Research Center found that people on the left and the right of political ideology have different notions about fake news. According to the study, fake news causes panic, and rather than uniting people with similar ideas, it drives them further to the fringe, polarizing them. As a result, customers will drop an outlet, people may cut out social relationships, and others reject any information on a specific topic. Believing in myths will have a similar result.

This is why it is essential to consider the truth about IF and read with as little bias as possible. The good news is that as powerful as misinformation is, truth is more powerful – it sets one free. In this chapter, I will explore the most common myths about IF and the truth about them so that you can be motivated as you look to make the necessary changes in your life.

Myth #1: Intermittent fasting is about starving yourself.

This myth is common among people new to IF and is spread by some who tried it for a day and gave up, probably due to the same misconception. As you fast, your body will start using energy differently. Rather than draw its energy from glucose, the body burns stored fat for energy, and ketosis occurs. You will not enter starvation mode during IF. The human body has evolved to go for short periods without food. Our ancestors did it, and so can we. Besides, studies show that fasting has many health benefits.

Myth #2: You are always stressed when you are fasting.

Proponents of this myth have learned to associate IF with stress. They probably carry false ideas from other diet plans that require you to do so much – count calories, weigh what you eat, meticulously track your weight, etc. They also imagine that your body is stressed because you go for some hours without food. This could not be further from the truth. Short-term fasting does not stress your body and has no impact on your stress hormone levels. Research has found that short-term fasting lowers your cortisol levels, regulates your immune system, metabolizes the fat in the body, and stabilizes your blood pressure.

Myth #3: It is impossible to focus while on IF.

Here, the idea is that you will feel hungry during fasting and therefore be unable to focus, making it hard for you to work. However, research does not support this idea. IF does not negatively affect your cognitive functions. If it did, why would so many religions in the world recommend fasting as a way to focus on their chosen deity? Studies show that short fasting periods have the opposite effect – improving cognitive function and stimulating better memory and faster learning.

Myth #4: You should always skip breakfast when on IF.

This is one of those dangerous types of misinformation that has some basis in the truth. Some people skip breakfast when doing IF, but you do not have to skip breakfast if that does not work for you. Every method of IF has different eating windows; you can choose an eating window that allows you to eat breakfast. IF is friendlier than other diets because it enables you to decide when to eat and plan according to your social events and hunger patterns.

I may as well address another breakfast-related myth now – the belief that breakfast is the most important meal of the day. How many times have you heard that said? Well, it stretches the truth too far. Eating when you wake up causes you to miss some of the benefits of extended fasting. However, even when you pick a fasting window that allows you to eat breakfast, it is always a good idea to break your fast with some water, wait about ten minutes and then eat.

Myth #5: All IF is the same and brings similar results.

Proponents of this myth believe that all people practicing IF do it the same way and will have the same results, but this is only partially true. The truth is that every person on a fast will go through the same stages/cycle, but that's where the similarities between IF methods and results end. There are different methods of IF. Time-restricted fasting, for example, splits your day between eating and fasting periods – you could eat for eight hours and fast for 16. Other methods use daily eating windows or require you to eat only one meal a day. Simply put, many fasting patterns fall under the umbrella of IF. Each person's body responds differently depending on their genetics, diet during non-fasting periods, and other factors like whether they exercise.

Myth #6: IF works for everyone.

We might think that because of its simplicity and health benefits, IF is suitable for everyone, but this is not the case. Intermittent fasting is not recommended for persons who have had an eating disorder in the past. It's also not a smart idea to attempt if you're pregnant, underweight, or frail. Breastfeeding mothers should not begin IF unless they are under the supervision of a doctor. Finally, during their developmental years, youngsters will not benefit from fasting. They need to eat to fuel their growth. To be safe, consult your doctor or a wellness expert before making any changes to your eating pattern.

Myth #7: During the eating window, you can eat as much of any food as you desire.

True, IF is adaptable and, compared to other diets, has the fewest food restrictions. The eating window, however, is not an excuse to make up for missing meals or indulge in harmful binges. That is the time to consume a healthy, well-balanced diet. Eat whole grains, healthy fats, lean proteins, veggies, and fruits in various combinations. If you still want something less healthy after that, go ahead and eat it, but don't overdo it. If you keep your food well-balanced and healthy during the eating window, you will get better results and find it easier to maintain IF.

Myth #8: IF causes your metabolism to slow down.

People believe intermittent fasting lowers their metabolism because of the fatigue they experience when fasting, particularly on the first or second day. Short-term fasting, such as the 16/8 technique, has the opposite impact— it boosts your metabolism and improves your adaptability. Fasting allows your body to rest, which is vital to benefit from metabolism-boosting hormonal and chemical changes. Besides, fasting causes your body to produce more hormonal regulators, such as the growth hormone and norepinephrine, which improve metabolism.

Myth #9: IF leads to overeating.

The idea here is that whenever people fast, they will overindulge as soon as they break their fast. This is not usually true. Research shows that as soon as people start seeing the benefits of IF, they get motivated to become more mindful of their eating. Little changes encourage them further as they accumulate and compound over time. For some people, it also works as part of a healthy long-term diet pattern. Because the eating window is timed, they learn to plan their meals and prepare before time, so they do not waste a lot of the eating window looking for what to eat.

Myth #10: You must reduce how much water you take as you fast.

Here, people are mistaken in assuming that water has calories too, and drinking during fasting beats the whole point of IF. However, this is not true. Restricting your water intake during fasts is not a good idea. In fact, you need to increase it. Water helps balance the acid levels in your body, regulate hormones and eliminate waste from your body.

Myth #11: IF does not help get rid of body toxins.

This is a myth most endorsed by the critics of IF. They find it difficult to see how fasting can help eliminate waste from the body, but the research is not on their side. One of the best things about IF is its ability to eliminate waste products in a process called autophagy. Autophagy is how cells clean out the accumulated dead cells in the body and has been linked to an extended lifespan. In a sense, fasting is a natural detox.

Myth #12: IF is unsustainable.

This is a common misconception among newbies – they wonder if they can keep up IF for the rest of their life. The answer is that it is up to you to decide. On its own, IF is very sustainable because it is not about restrictions like other diets. In fact, IF does away with the mentality that demands you constantly deny yourself certain foods – the diet mentality. With IF, it is easy to control your intake without constantly battling your cravings. Once you set a schedule and get used to it, you only have to think about food when it is time to eat, and when that time comes, you can enjoy your food and eat healthy portions. IF even allows you to have a social life – you can plan your eating window around when you will be around others. The diet's flexibility makes it sustainable.

Myth #13: You cannot exercise while you are fasting.

Some people imagine it will be challenging to work out on IF, but that is an unfounded fear. Instead, it is recommended that you include exercise as part of your lifestyle to boost your metabolism and burn fat faster. Besides that, research shows that the best time to work out is when your stomach is empty because your body will draw on fat for fuel, helping you burn more calories than you would have otherwise burned.

Myth #14: You can become incredibly fit through fasting alone.

IF is an excellent eating pattern for weight loss. It also has many benefits for your health, but IF alone cannot make you fit. Combining IF with proper exercise is the best way to lose weight more effectively and become fit. It is exercise that will improve your flexibility and balance, not fasting. So, the rumors are untrue – IF on its own is not the magic solution that will make you fit. You will need to develop other habits to help you maintain your ideal weight, but it comes closer than many other diets.

Myth #15: IF works because your body does not process food at night.

This is a significant misconception about how fasting works. People imagine digestion does not happen when you are asleep, but this is not true. Your body digests food regardless of the time and whether you are resting or in motion. IF is more about giving your body enough time to digest food and focus on other metabolic processes like cellular repair and autophagy.

There could be other misconceptions about fasting within the health and fitness community, but this chapter debunks the most common myths. You are now better equipped to decide how to add IF to your lifestyle. The next chapter will further educate you by answering the commonly asked questions about intermittent fasting.

Chapter 5
The Intermittent FAQ

I n the previous chapter, we discussed how you cannot become fit just by fasting, how sustainable IF is, and how you can include breakfast in your IF schedule if that's what you want. The idea? To demystify some of the myths connected to IF. It is clear that if you are going to change to an IF lifestyle, you need to do some research and learn enough to know precisely what you are getting yourself into. For instance, did you know that IF is not really a diet? Many people imagine it is because you skip meals, but technically, a diet is not a diet because you skip a meal. The primary characteristic of a diet is that you are told what to eat. IF tells you when you can eat. How sweet is that!

Besides, IF not only tells you when you can eat, it gives you options for how you approach your food. If you are still convinced that breakfast is the most important meal of the day, you can have an excellent breakfast and go on with your IF plan. If you feel it is vital to eat lunch, then have lunch. It is a lot like shopping for clothes –there are options for everyone. IF is more accurately an eating schedule than a diet, but it can help with weight loss. You will be eating within a selected time frame, which means you eat less than you typically do, reducing your calorie intake. As a result, you lose weight.

And in addition to its weight loss benefits, IF helps keep your hormones happy. Do you know the feeling when you finally have a few days off work after a crazy schedule? That is how your body feels when you give it a break from digesting food for a while. First, it focuses on keeping your cells and hormones healthy and happy instead of only breaking down food. That's when your insulin levels drop while your growth hormone levels increase. That change alone boosts the fat-burning process in your body. Secondly, your body ramps up autophagy, an action that promotes weight management and anti-aging. Finally, fasting changes gene expression, protecting you from serious diseases in the future.

Of course, with all these benefits, it is worth mentioning that you need to break your fast in the correct way. The right way to break your fast involves drinking a lot of water. Ideally, you were also drinking water during your fast. But when breaking it, it is particularly important to drink water or a warm beverage that will stimulate diges-tion when you start eating. If you prefer, drink ginger tea or lemon water. Eat fruit as well. During fasting, your body interacts with your glycogen stores as during an intense workout. Eating fruit gives your body natural sugars to refill your glycogen stores. There is a lot to process about IF. Here are some commonly asked questions and their answers:

Question #1: How does IF differ from dieting?

During IF, you alternate between eating periods and fasting periods, resulting in a significant decrease in your calorie intake. Most diets focus on what you eat, not when you eat. IF is not cutting out or depriving yourself of certain foods. It is about eating during a specific time and then fasting for the rest of the time.

Question #2: How does intermittent fasting really work?

There are different versions of IF, including the 16/8, 5/2, and alternate-day fasting and their derivatives. In the 16/8 fasting method, you fast for 16 hours and have an 8-hour eating window. It is time-restricted. The alternate-day fasting approach involves limiting your calories on fasting days and eating normally on alternating days. The 5/2 fasting method means fasting for two non-consecutive days a week and eating without restrictions during the other five. Every version of IF involves restricting your food intake or avoiding it altogether for a certain period.

Question #3: Are the benefits of intermittent fasting real?

IF has many suggested benefits that are supported by research and anecdotal evidence. First, *Current Obesity Reports* show that IF is linked to weight loss. Data suggest a weight loss of between 5 and 9.9 percent within the first month of starting. Research from *Nutrition and Healthy Aging* supports these findings. Secondly, according to a study published in *Cell*, IF is said to lengthen life. The researchers used a lab model to look at cell aging markers and observed how they behaved under calorie restriction. Restricting calories helped reduce inflammation and slow the aging process. However, more of this kind of research is needed.

Thirdly, IF reduces insulin resistance, a condition common in type 2 diabetes patients. The CDC supports this, adding that it does so by reducing calorie intake. Fourthly, according to a study published by the *Nutrition Journal*, IF improves heart health. Researchers observed that participants in the study lost weight and burnt fat through intermittent fasting. Finally, IF results in healthier metabolic markers and enhanced memory. A study done in 2021 and published in *Molecular Psychiatry* found that IF worked better than traditional diets at enhancing memory and improving metabolic markers. All the benefits of IF are backed by science, but the extent to which every person experiences them varies based on genetics, diet, and consistency.

Question #4: When should I start fasting?

There is no clear-cut time when you can start fasting, but there are some indicators that can tell you when the time is right. First, you need to have a health goal. Do you know what you hope to accomplish with fasting? Is it weight loss? Is it a generally healthier lifestyle? Decide on why you need IF. When you have that answer, talk to your primary caregiver. Your doctor will help you decide whether IF is good for your body. Ask them all the questions you may have about the eating plan and how it will affect your body.

Finally, choose the best IF approach for you. Look at the way you socialize and how your daily tasks are organized. Which IF method will best complement your lifestyle? Remember that it is okay to experiment with different fasting windows to determine what works for you. Once you are familiar with the basics of IF, you can start fasting.

Question #5: When did intermittent fasting start?

People have been fasting for millennia. The *Academy of Nutrition and Dietetics Journal* says that ancient religions were the first to practice voluntary and intentional fasting. Back then, fasting was a way to regulate the body and submit to a better spiritual life. However, the version of IF used today is about ten years old. Harvard Health says that IF became popular in 2012 after the documentary *Eat, Fast and Live Longer* went live. A little research shows that many books about the fasting method were published around that period. Heavy research followed over the next five years.

Question #6: Are there certain people who can't do intermittent fasting? Who are they?

Health professionals recommend that some people avoid IF or do it only under a doctor's supervision. IF may not be for you if you have type 1 diabetes, for example, or if you have type 2 diabetes and on insulin prescription. It improves insulin sensitivity but will not help you if you take medications associated with low blood sugar. IF is also not recommended if you have a chronic illness. There is limited research about how the eating plan affects other diseases, but adverse side effects like dizziness could be worse for sick people. Be careful not to aggravate your medical issues by failing to eat regularly. If you are on medication for heart disease, you will likely be more affected by the electrolyte imbalances associated with fasting, so IF may not be a good idea.

Other than those, do not attempt IF if you are underweight or have a history of eating disorders. If your BMI is below 18.5, IF will do more harm than good. If you have disordered eating, IF will make your relationship with food more unhealthy. Generally speaking, consult with a doctor before you start fasting whether or not you suffer from any of these conditions. Lastly, IF is not recommended for pregnant or breastfeeding women. Research has proven that breastfeeding is not the best time to reduce calorie intake because women need to sustain milk production and keep their energy levels high.

Question #7: How best do you break a fast?

The end of your fasting period should not be an excuse to binge on unhealthy foods – if you do that, it will undermine your success. The principles of healthy eating still apply even when you are on IF. Focus on eating a balanced diet. Be particularly careful to eat a lot of protein if you have diabetes. Protein does not break down into glucose the same way carbs will, so it will have a less immediate effect on your blood sugar levels. That said, break your fast with water or a warm beverage. It will help your body prepare to digest food once you start eating.

Question #8: Can I exercise while I'm intermittent fasting?

Yes. You can exercise while doing IF. Research suggests that exercising during the fasted state will help you burn fat. The body needs sugar to sustain your exercise. Typically, it gets that energy from glycogen in the liver. When you exercise during the fasted state, those glycogen stores are already depleted, so the body finds an alternative energy source. It resorts to an anaerobic breakdown of fat to give you energy.

Question #9: Can intermittent fasting really help me lose weight?

The short answer to this question is yes. IF is an excellent tool for weight management and weight loss. It helps you lose weight because you go for long periods between meals, which allows the body to use stored fat in the cells for energy. During this period, your insulin levels reduce. Remember that any weight loss comes about because of calorie restriction. In general, people gain weight because they eat more calories than they are burning and lose weight because they eat less than they are burning. Of course, other factors like diet and genetics play a role, but generally, weight loss is governed by this principle.

IF helps you lose weight because it gives you a smaller eating window compared to eating the whole day. Research published by the *Nutrition and Healthy Aging Journal* showed that twenty-three obese adults reduced their calorie intake by about 300 calories a day when they attempted 16/8 IF. Time-restricted fasting can also help you eliminate eating habits that do not support weight loss – such as nighttime snacking.

Question #10: How can I control my hunger during my fasting?

The chances are that you will feel hungry, especially in the initial stages as your body adjusts to IF. However, it gets easier as time goes on. One way to deal with the hunger, though, is to integrate IF into your lifestyle and your schedule. First, do not make drastic changes at once. For example, if you start work at 8 a.m. and you have a demanding job, you can arrange to have a fasting window that allows you breakfast. Secondly, during the fasting period, try to stay engaged. If you let your mind dwell on food, you will become hungrier and more likely to cave in. Thirdly, keep hydrating. Drinking water during your fasting window can help to suppress hunger. It tricks the body into thinking it's fuller, allowing you to fast more comfortably.

Question #11: Is there a right way to fast?

IF is popular because it does not dictate what you eat as other diets do. This means that there is no right way to fast, as long as you abide by the general principle of the diet – have a fasting and an eating window. Even so, there are different types of IF, including the 5/2 diet, 16/8, 14/10, alternate-day, and eat-stop-eat fasting. Choose the approach that works well with your lifestyle and preferences, and it will be the right way for you to fast.

Question #12: Can intermittent fasting really help me?

Yes. Intermittent fasting can really help you. Whenever you fast, your body starts getting energy from ketones rather than glucose in a metabolic switching process. Changes occur in your body with autophagy which makes it possible for you to lose weight. It also has other longer-lasting health benefits such as reduced inflammation, increased energy levels, improved sleep patterns, improved digestion, and a strengthened immune system. Remember that in some cases, you will experience only one or two of those health benefits because everyone's metabolism works differently, and you may need to eat more than someone else.

Generally speaking, though, fasting helps some people to feel more energetic while others struggle to adjust. If IF does not make you feel better mentally or physically after the first week, consult with a health professional. It takes a maximum of a week for your body to adapt to new eating habits. Any side effects should disappear after a week.

Question #13: Can you really lose weight eating the same amount but changing the times you eat?

Not really, but it depends. Weight loss results from a caloric deficit. Your body needs to be getting fewer calories than it is burning for you to lose weight. You may see minimal weight loss results if you practice IF but still eat the same amount. This is because your body will take considerable time digesting the food you ate before it resorts to the fat reservoirs. There will be a very short fat-burning window before the next eating period. It is worth noting that most people naturally change their eating habits and the quantities they eat when they start IF. After trying the eating plan for a couple of weeks and seeing the results, they are motivated to make little changes, which multiply and lead to a healthier lifestyle.

Question #14: What concerns do some dieticians have about intermittent fasting?

Dieticians fear that people may not know enough to balance their diet when it comes to IF. During IF or any diet plan involving calorie restriction, you need to have a well-balanced diet that gives you the nutrients you need every day. No one should risk nutrient deficiencies, whether or not you are fasting.

Question #15: Does intermittent fasting come with side effects?

Yes, IF has some side effects such as hunger, cravings, lightheadedness, headaches, irritability, and other mood changes, all connected to the hormonal changes associated with fasting. Most people experience them in the initial days of fasting, but after a maximum of seven days, your body adjusts to the new eating pattern.

Question #16: Are some types of intermittent fasting more effective than others?

Different types of IF work in different ways for different people, but no one method is more effective than the other. Fasting works the same way as our regular eating habits — they work differently for different people.

Question #17: Can I still eat three meals during intermittent fasting?

You can still eat three meals daily during IF, but you must do it mindfully. Some people combine breakfast and lunch when they break their fast and then include snacks within their day. At night, they end their eating period with a light dinner. Be sure to pick foods that are heavy on protein and fiber as they are more filling.

Question #18: Why am I still gaining weight when intermittent fasting?

If you start IF and notice you are gaining weight, it could be that you are eating too many calories during your eating period. If you overeat during the eating window to try to make up for the period you are fasting, it will not work. The types of food you eat also count – high-calorie foods will undoubtedly cause you to gain weight rather than lose it.

You could also be gaining weight because you are not eating enough. If you do not eat enough food during your eating period, you increase the likelihood that you will binge-eat during the next window because you are starving. This is because you will be so hungry that you do not stop when you start eating. No wonder fasting is not recommended for people who have a disordered eating pattern. It can lead you into an unhealthy pattern that leaves you worse off.

The third reason you may be gaining weight is that you are probably not eating enough protein. Regardless of the type of IF you pick, you need protein. That protein could come from chicken, lean meat, or protein powders. It helps build muscle mass, fosters bone health, and helps you recover after exercise.

As you can see, some things about IF are different from what people think. However, you now have all the information you need for your intermittent fasting journey. The next chapter will suggest a few lifestyle changes and start you on your IF journey.

Chapter 6
The Lifestyle Change

More and more people are embracing the different types of IF. They are starting to accept that when you eat has a bearing on weight loss. A major social media network CEO hit the headlines recently when he announced that he eats only one meal a day. Some people thought his diet plan was extreme, while others celebrated his efforts. Last year, the International Food Information Council confirmed that IF is currently the most popular diet.

One of the main reasons IF is so popular is its structure. People do not like to be told just to eat a healthy and balanced diet. They prefer a bit more structure, and IF gives them that. It allows them to be disciplined in their eating patterns without the strict policing that is typical of other diets. IF does not restrict certain food groups like carbs, sugars, or fats. All you need is to focus on when to eat rather than what to eat. Perhaps that is the eating pattern's biggest appeal. Most people who come to the diet do so because it is simple to adopt. With small steps, you can change your lifestyle and eating patterns. This chapter is about that. It is about integrating the changes you need to make to live a healthier life.

Making the Shift

So far, you have learned what constitutes IF, the different types, and their benefits. In addition, we have demystified some of the misinformation about eating patterns. The previous chapter answered some common questions. Hopefully, you are excited to start the diet now that you have the science at your fingertips. The next question is: why should your commitment to a healthy lifestyle change include IF?

First of all, IF will help you with weight loss. Most people who practice this method lose weight and lose it fast. This is because, with IF, you eat fewer calories, lose fat, and boost your metabolism. Secondly, IF will lower your risk of type 2 diabetes; it reduces your insulin resistance and blood sugar levels. Finally, embracing IF will improve your health in general. It will increase your heart health and may help prevent diseases like cancer and Alzheimer's.

In simple terms, IF can help you reach your health goals no matter how different they are from the next person's. The natural calorie restrictions involved in IF will help you lose weight without the complications of a strict diet. You do not have to keep counting calories or worry about cooking three meals a day. You only have to think about food during the eating period.

IF can be difficult for some at the beginning. Some women experience headaches when starting the program. Others become irritable. However, this does not have to be you. You do not need to torture yourself to live healthily. Instead, start making changes slowly. No step is too small. For example, if you eat three times a day at the moment, you can start by eliminating your in-between-meals snacks. Alternatively, you can reduce your eating window by ten minutes. Do not be over-ambitious. Be happy to take small but steady steps until you have made the necessary adjustments. Use the following steps to get started:

Step 1: Pick your method

As you have seen in this book, there are various intermittent fasting methods. Go back to Chapter two and study them. Which one is best suited to you and your schedule? That is the one for you.

Step 2: Think about your meals

After picking the method that suits you, decide beforehand what you will eat. If you can, prepare some meals. If that is not possible, simply plan what you will eat. That way, you will not waste time obsessing over food.

Step 3: Take baby steps

The journey of a thousand miles starts with one step. Do not expect your body to get accustomed to fasting immediately. That is unreasonable. Instead, make minor adjustments to what you eat and when you eat to work your way up to your chosen method of IF. For instance, if you prefer the 5/2 pattern but have a hard time fasting for 24 hours, begin with eight hours or less and then work upward.

Step 4: Exercise

Exercise increases your metabolism, boosting fat burning and weight loss. It also triggers happy hormones, so you feel more cheerful. So include some exercise in your lifestyle.

The Gradual Approach

Take the gradual approach when starting IF. This means starting slowly, in small incremental steps that are easy to make and maintain. Its core philosophy is making things as simple as possible to increase the likelihood that you not only make the shift but also stick with it. It consists of the following pillars:

1. Eat your dinner early.

The first principle of the gradual approach is that you should not eat for at least three hours before going to bed.

This is because your sleep hormone levels increase in the evening as you approach bedtime. That hormone, melatonin, is connected to high body fat and body mass index. This is the science behind the principle of eating early. Three hours may seem a lot, but you can work toward that target slowly. Start by identifying when you are comfortable eating dinner and how long that is from your bedtime. Then, eat fifteen minutes earlier and keep at it until you adjust. Keep doing that until you are comfortable, and then move your dinner time forward by another fifteen minutes. Keep doing that until you eat at least three hours before bed.

The other scientific reason behind eating early is the impact of insulin on growth hormone production. The growth hormone is produced within your first hours of sleep. It helps with endocrine function, cell repair, and healthy metabolism. If its production is dysregulated, you experience hormonal imbalance. You risk getting sick and gaining weight when your hormones are not functioning correctly. Besides that, cell repair and detox happen at night. If your body is too busy digesting food, it will not have enough time to perform cell repair.

2. Increase the periods between your meals.

You can extend the period before eating slowly so that you never feel anxious about it or irritable due to hunger. As a side note, ensure that all the meals you eat have the nutrients your body needs to fuel you for your day's activities. It does not have to be a feast, but every meal needs proteins, healthy fats, and vegetables. These foods get digested slowly, so you will not experience an immediate spike in your insulin levels. High blood insulin levels translate to hunger and sugar cravings.

When implementing this principle, you may find it hard to go for long periods without food. That's okay. Take your minimum period, say three hours, and increase it by ten or fifteen minutes. Practice that until you can extend the interval without punishing yourself. The goal is to be able to go six hours before your next meal. Your increased duration should match an increase in macronutrient ratios and quantity. Experiment as much as you need to until you learn to listen to and understand your body. With time, you will enjoy the benefits of fat adaptation, including better performance, increased energy, and improved mental clarity.

3. Remove your focus from calorie restriction.

As you adjust your eating window, do not cut down on how much you eat. IF is not an excuse to starve yourself. Restricting calories greatly will lower your metabolic rate and work against your goal. You will feel hungrier later on and will struggle to fast. Do not make the process harder than it should be.

4. Break your fast mindfully.

After many hours of not eating, ensure that the first meal you eat sets you up for a successful day. Eat healthy fats, whole-plant fiber, and protein. Ideally, the meal should also include some Omega-3 fats. Do not break your fast with foods high in carbohydrates, whether cereals, muffins, or bread. These will spike your leptin levels early in the day and make you feel hungry sooner. If you anticipate being too busy to make a proper meal when breaking your fast, you can prepare your meal in advance or lengthen your fast to allow time to make a good meal. You can also make a smoothie to get you started as you cook. Just do not binge on carbohydrates.

As you implement these principles, your body will start adjusting to eating less. When you notice the change, you can begin reorganizing your meals to either eat later or stop eating earlier, depending on your preferred IF method. Remember to always focus on timing rather than calorie restriction and let the rest fall into place. Some days will be more challenging than others, but that's part of the process. Stick with it, and you will be glad you did when you start seeing the results.

Tips to Get Started

Tip #1: Be guided by your schedule

Keep your schedule in mind as you figure out which IF type is best for you. You should not select an IF type simply because it is popular or because someone you know has done it. If your schedule is so unpredictable that you can't eat all your meals in eight hours, the 16/8 may not be the ideal solution for you. If you can't go twenty-four hours without eating, the eat-stop-eat method isn't for you. Consider your lifestyle and whether the plan you choose will impact the people in your life. The shift will be smoother if it fits your schedule.

Tip #2: Figure out when best to do your workout

While it is true that you can exercise while on IF, you must figure out when to do it so that you are not too hungry to exercise effectively, especially at the beginning. The best time to work out is early in the morning. Exercise will revitalize you and regulate your hormones. Evening and afternoon workouts demand more from you because you are fatigued from the day and coping with whatever pressures have come your way. Even so, exercising at this time of day is still possible.

Tip #3: Do not forget your goal as you eat

After you've determined when to eat and when to fast, the next step is to decide what to consume during the eating window. The rule is to eat with your objective in mind. Limit your carbohydrate intake if you want to lose weight. You can prepare healthy low-carb meals ahead of time so you are not tempted to pick up the next available carb when you break your fast. Focus on vegetables and lean protein. If you're fasting for general health reasons, stick to whole food. Avoid processed foods and check the labels on the foods you buy to avoid eating too much added sugar. Balance healthy fats, vegetables, and proteins in your meals.

Tip #4: Have no cheat days

For most people, a cheat day is a day when they binge eat and indulge in all of their cravings. However, the consequences of that binge last longer than twenty-four hours. Recovery, regaining focus and energy, and controlling cravings might take up to four days. Having a cheat day is not worth it. IF aims to get you to your health goal as quickly as possible. A cheat day will simply throw you off track or make you abandon your goal. Even so, eating a piece of cake or some ice cream occasionally is okay.

Tip #5: Stay hydrated

During IF, you cannot possibly drink too much water. Drink plenty of water or calorie-free beverages like herbal teas and sugarless coffee to stay hydrated throughout the day.

Tip #6: Remove any tempting treats from your home.

If you're fasting to lose weight, your meals should be high in protein and vegetables. You'll lose sight of your goals if you eat random chocolate bars, biscuits, cupcakes, and other carbohydrate-based snacks. When you first start IF, get rid of them so they don't become an unwanted temptation.

As you make these adjustments, give yourself time to grow to love your new habits. Change things one at a time to avoid feeling overwhelmed. Over the following few chapters, I will provide a complete list of exciting breakfast, lunch, and dinner recipes to help you eat healthily.

Chapter 7
The Recipes - Breakfast

Breakfast is the most controversial meal when it comes to IF. Many people believe breakfast is the most important meal of the day, so they cannot imagine skipping it. However, conversely, other people think skipping breakfast is essential. The second group of people wonders how they can lose weight while still consuming those breakfast calories. The truth lies between these two extremes – deciding whether you eat breakfast during IF is your choice.

It is worth remembering that skipping breakfast, especially when you are transitioning from a lifestyle where you ate every meal, might work against you. It would be best to have breakfast to keep your metabolism working smoothly after a long all-night fast. Eating breakfast is not always about your weight. It is about minerals, vitamins, protein, and muscle mass. It is about eating healthy to make your body feel good and function as it should. It is about the nutritional content of your food.

One of the things people come to love about IF is that they enjoy their food when it is finally breakfast time. This is why, after so many hours without food, you do not want to just down a cup of coffee and a protein bar and get on with your day. Instead, you want a breakfast that you can savor. You want recipes that will make your mouth water and satisfy your taste buds and hunger. This is what this chapter is for. Here, I provide recipes for every season, whether you are busy and have a few minutes to whip up a meal or have time to prepare something more elaborate. Some recipes are excellent to make ahead of time, while others work when you are extremely busy.

▷ Turkish eggs

Servings: 2 (469 calories per serving)

Total time: 13 minutes

Ingredients:

- 5 large eggs
- 2 tablespoons olive oil
- 1 whole-wheat pita
- 2 tablespoons plain yogurt
- ¾ cup diced red bell pepper
- ¾ cup diced eggplant
- Pepper and salt to taste

- Cilantro, chopped to taste
- ¼ teaspoon paprika

Directions

1. Heat a pan and pour oil. Add bell pepper, eggplant, salt and pepper. Cook for seven minutes until soft.
2. Add eggs, paprika, salt and pepper to taste. Keep stirring for two more minutes.
3. Spice with cilantro and serve with the pita and yogurt.

▷ Chickpea waffles

Servings: 2 (412 calories per serving)

Total time: 20 minutes

Ingredients

- ¾ cup chickpea flour
- Pepper and salt to taste
- ½ teaspoon baking soda
- ¾ cup plain Greek yogurt
- 6 large eggs
- olive oil, cucumbers, and tomatoes for serving

Directions

1. Preheat the oven to 190°C. Set your waffle iron as per its directions and preheat it. Coat it with cooking spray.
2. Whisk the flour, baking soda, and salt in a bowl. Mix the egg and yogurt in a different bowl and pour them into the flour mix.
3. Pour the mix into the waffle iron in batches of ¼ cup each. Cook for four minutes or until golden brown. Transfer the waffles into the oven to keep warm, and repeat the process until you finish the batter.
4. Serve waffles with tomatoes, cucumbers, and olive oil.

▷ Scrambled egg and sweet potatoes

This is an excellent recipe for days when you have only about 30 minutes to spare. You can prepare the sweet potatoes before time so that all you need to do in the morning is toss them in the oven.

Servings: 1 (571 calories)

Total time: 25 minutes

Ingredients

- 1 piece diced sweet potato
- ½ cup chopped onion
- 2 teaspoons chopped rosemary
- 4 large eggs
- 4 large egg whites
- 2 tablespoons chopped chives

Directions

1. Preheat your oven to 220°C. Combine the chopped sweet potato with the spices and lay them on a baking sheet. Use cooking spray and roast for 20 minutes until tender.
2. Whisk the eggs and egg whites in a bowl and season with pepper and salt. Scramble them in a skillet for 5 minutes as it roasts.
3. Sprinkle the eggs with chives and serve with sweet potatoes.

▷ Cabbage scramble and egg

This recipe is suitable for days you have only a few minutes to spare. Both eggs and cabbage cook quickly. You can pre-chop the cabbage and eggs and refrigerate them until you need to use them.

Servings: 1 (400 Calories)

Total time: 10 minutes

Ingredients

- ½ tablespoon organic butter
- 2 scrambled eggs
- ½ cup sliced onions
- 2 cups chopped cabbage
- Salt to taste

Directions

1. Put some butter on a pan and sauté the cabbage and onions for five minutes. Salt and plate.
2. Use the remaining butter to cook your eggs. Top with the pumpkin seeds and serve with the cabbage.

▷ Strawberry chia bowl with coconut

Servings: 1 (200 calories)

Total time: 35 minutes

Ingredients

- 2 tablespoons unsweetened coconut flakes
- 2 tablespoons chia seeds
- 4 tablespoons cashews
- ¼ cup organic Greek yogurt
- ¼ cup unsweetened coconut milk

- ¼ cup unsweetened almond butter (or peanut butter)
- ½ cup sliced strawberries

Directions

1. Mix the Greek yogurt, coconut milk, and chia seeds in a bowl. Let them sit for 30 minutes.
2. Top with the rest of the ingredients and serve. You can store extra servings in the fridge for up to three days or freeze them for two weeks.

▷ Parmesan and spinach breakfast

Servings: 1 (354 calories)

Total time: 7 minutes

Ingredients

- 2 free-range eggs
- 1 tablespoon olive oil
- Salt and black pepper to taste
- 2 cups washed baby spinach
- 1 clove garlic, crushed
- 3 tablespoons Parmesan cheese, grated

Directions

1. In a pan, fry the garlic for 30 seconds in the olive oil. Keep stirring it to avoid browning.
2. Add the spinach and salt it. It may look like you have too much spinach, but it will wilt and reduce as you keep stirring.
3. Whisk the eggs in a bowl as the spinach cooks, and add half of the parmesan and black pepper. Pour them over the spinach and stir for 40 seconds or until the eggs set. Do not overcook them, or they will be dry. Remove the eggs after a minute, and they will continue cooking without the heat.
4. Scatter the remaining parmesan and serve.

▷ Buttered Oats and Jelly

Servings: 1 (255 calories)

Total time: 5 minutes (without counting refrigeration time)

Ingredients

- ½ cup 2% milk
- ¼ cup rolled oats
- ¼ cup raspberries, mashed and 3 tablespoons whole berries
- Peanut butter

Directions

1. Mix the peanut butter, mashed raspberries, milk, and oats in a bowl. Stir to form a smooth mixture.
2. Refrigerate overnight. During breakfast, top with the whole raspberries and serve.

▷ Avocado and cheese toast

Servings: 1 (288 calories)

Total time: 5 minutes

Ingredients

- 1 slice whole-grain bread
- ¼ smashed avocado
- 2 tablespoons ricotta cheese
- Salt to taste
- Red pepper flakes as desired

Directions

1. Toast your slice of bread the way you like it.
2. Top with avocado, ricotta, and red pepper flakes. Season with salt and serve with scrambled eggs.

▷ Tofu scramble

Servings: 1 (431 calories)

Total time: 15 minutes

Ingredients

- ½ sliced avocado, sliced
- Pepper and salt to taste
- 4 cherry tomatoes
- 1 portabella mushroom
- ½ block firm Tofu
- 2 tablespoons olive oil
- ¼ teaspoon ground turmeric
- Garlic powder to taste

Directions

1. Preheat the oven to 220°C. Lay the mushroom and tomatoes on a baking sheet and brush them with half of the olive oil. Season to taste with pepper and salt. Roast for ten minutes.
2. Combine tofu, turmeric, garlic, and salt in a bowl as the mushroom and tomatoes roast. Mash them.
3. Put a large skillet over medium heat, add the remaining olive oil, and heat. Pour the tofu mixture into the skillet and cook for three minutes until it becomes firm. Keep stirring.
4. Serve the tofu with the tomatoes, mushrooms, and avocado.

▷ **Blueberry smoothie**

Servings: 1 (256 calories)

Total time: 5 minutes (without counting freezing time)

Ingredients

- ½ frozen banana
- 1 ½ cups unsweetened coconut milk (or water, or almond milk)
- 2 tablespoons chia seeds
- ¾ cup unsweetened Greek yogurt
- 2 tablespoons almond (or peanut) butter
- ¼ cup frozen blueberries

Directions

1. Blend all the ingredients until smooth.
2. Serve. You can top it with cacao nibs if you like.

▷ **Almond muffins**

Servings: 5 (484 calories per serving)

Total time: 15 minutes

Ingredients

- ½ stick butter
- 1 tablespoon cinnamon
- 1 tablespoon allspice

- 2 cups almond meal
- 4 large eggs
- 4 scoops vanilla protein powder
- 1 cup unsweetened applesauce
- 2 teaspoons baking powder
- 1 teaspoon cloves

Directions

1. Preheat the oven to 180°C. Melt the butter on low heat until fully melted.
2. Mix the rest of the ingredients into the butter and prepare muffin tins.
3. Pour the batter into the tins to ¾ full. You should use about ten muffins.
4. Bake for 12 minutes. If you bake them for longer, they will be too dry. Serve warm.

▷ The green smoothie

Servings: 1 (256 calories)

Total time: 5 minutes

Ingredients

- 1 cup spinach
- ½ cup frozen pineapple
- 1 cup water
- 1 banana

- ½ cup frozen mango

Directions

1. Pour spinach and the water into a blender. Blend until smooth.
2. Add the other ingredients and blend to get a smooth and creamy mix. It will take up to two minutes, depending on your blender.
3. Serve immediately, or store it covered in the fridge until you are ready to serve.

▷ Peanut Butter and Chia jam sandwich

Servings: 2 (300 calories per serving)

Total time: 35 minutes

Ingredients

- ½ cup raspberries
- 8 large brown rice cakes
- ½ cup blueberries
- 2 teaspoons honey
- 1 tablespoon chia seeds
- 4 tablespoons peanut butter
- ½ small apple cubed

Directions

1. Mix the chia seeds, blueberries, honey, raspberries, and a tablespoon of water in a bowl. Smash them until they look like jam.
2. Cover and refrigerate until the chia seeds become soft and the jam thickens - no more than 30 minutes.
3. Spread a rice cake with peanut butter and top with a quarter of the jam and some apple pieces. Cover with another sandwich and repeat to make three more. Two sandwiches make one serving.

Chapter 8 will provide a complete list of lunch recipes for days when you are busy and want a quick fix and some for those days you can afford to linger in the kitchen.

Chapter 8
The Recipes - Lunch

"Fasting is a lot like spring cleaning for your body."

— Jentezen Franklin

D o you occasionally have to go to an office where there is no microwave? No problem. There are recipes you can use for a cold lunch. Do you need something you can whip up quickly? That is covered too. In this chapter, you will find lunch recipes you can serve in different situations, from simple salads to spicy burritos to make your lunch worth the wait, refreshing, and healthy.

▷ Kale salad with Quinoa

Servings: 2 (512 calories per serving)

Total time: 45 minutes

Ingredients

- ½ cup tomato juice
- 1/8 teaspoon pepper
- 1 ½ cups water
- 1 cup quinoa, rinsed
- ¼ teaspoon salt
- 1 small onion, chopped
- 1 teaspoon lemon juice
- 1 tablespoon balsamic vinegar
- 1 teaspoon lemon zest, grated
- 1 tablespoon olive oil
- ¼ cup sunflower kernels – (you can also use pine nuts)
- ¼ cup cranberries – (you can replace with raisins)
- ½ teaspoon red pepper, crushed and flaked
- 1 garlic clove, minced
- 6 cups fresh kale, chopped

Directions

1. Mix the tomato juice and water in a pan and boil. Add the quinoa and reduce the heat. Cover and simmer until all the liquid is absorbed. It should take about 20 minutes. Switch off the heat and fluff the mixture using a fork.

2. Sauté the onion in the olive oil in a skillet until it becomes tender. Add the red pepper flakes and garlic and cook for another 45 seconds more.

3. Add kale while stirring and cook until the kale wilts. It should not take more than four minutes. Add the cranberries and sunflower kernels and cook for two more minutes.

4. Add the lemon zest, juice, and vinegar, and season with pepper and salt. Cook for two minutes and remove from heat.

5. Stir the quinoa into the kale and serve warm.

▷ Vegetable burritos

Servings: 4 (334 calories per serving)

Total time: 30 minutes

Ingredients

- 1 garlic clove, minced
- 1 bunch cilantro, chopped
- 1 cup white rice
- ½ teaspoon chipotle chili powder
- 1 cup black bean soup
- Kosher salt to taste
- 1 cup spinach, chopped
- 2 tablespoons lime juice
- 2 cups fire-roasted corn
- 1 large tomato, diced

- 4 flour tortillas
- 2 cups Jack cheese, shredded

Directions

1. Set aside three tablespoons of cilantro in a bowl. Mix the rest with two cups of water, ½ teaspoon salt, garlic, and chili powder in a blender, and puree until smooth. Transfer the blend to a saucepan, add the rice, and boil. Once it has boiled, set the heat to low and cook for 18 minutes or until the rice absorbs all the liquid. Stir and leave it to cool.

2. In a different pan, simmer the black bean soup and cook for three minutes. Add the spinach and simmer for two more minutes. Cover to keep them warm.

3. Mix the three tablespoons of cilantro, lime juice, corn, and tomato in a bowl. Add chili powder and salt to taste.

4. Use a microwave to warm the tortillas. Divide the mixtures into the tortillas in your preferred order. Add the corn salsa as a topping. Fold the bottoms, roll up the sides and serve the rest of the corn salsa. Serve.

▷ Tofu with roasted vegetables

Servings: 2 (454 calories per serving)

Total time: 10 minutes

Ingredients

- ½ cup cooked brown rice
- 1 cup roasted vegetables
- 1 cup roasted tofu
- 2 tablespoon scallions, sliced
- 2 tablespoons fresh cilantro, chopped
- 2 tablespoon cashew sauce

Directions

1. Arrange the tofu, vegetables, and rice in a bowl.
2. Sprinkle with the cilantro and scallions and serve with the cashew sauce.

▷ Tuna salad

Servings: 4 (172kcal per serving)

Total time: 15 minutes

Ingredients

- 2 cans tuna
- ½ tablespoon Dijon mustard
- ¼ cup mayonnaise
- 2 tablespoons red onion, diced
- 1 stalk celery, diced

- 2 tablespoons parsley – (you can also use another herb of choice)
- Pepper and salt to taste

Directions

1. Dry the tuna.
2. In a mixing bowl, add the celery, mustard, herbs, red onion, mayonnaise, and tuna, and stir. Season with pepper and salt to taste.
3. Serve plain or with lettuce.

▷ Rice salad seasoned with lemon and herbs

Servings: 6 (378 calories per serving)

Total Time: 50 minutes

Ingredients

- 2 lemons
- 1 bunch of watercress, with stems removed
- ½ cup basil, chopped
- pepper and salt to taste
- ½ cup mint, chopped
- ½ cup cilantro, chopped
- ½ red onion, medium, sliced
- ½ cup peanuts, roasted
- 1 cucumber, seeded and diced
- 1 carrot, shredded

- 2 teaspoons brown sugar
- 2 teaspoons rice wine vinegar
- 2 cups long-grain white rice
- ¼ cup vegetable oil

Directions

1. Use a vegetable peeler to cut two wide lemon zest strips from one lemon. Add one of the strips to the oil in a saucepan and cook until its edges become golden. It should take five minutes. Leave to cool.
2. As you wait, cook rice per its directions and add the other lemon strip to the water. When the rice is ready, put it in a bowl and remove the zest. Fluff it and leave it to cool.
3. Put the remaining lemons in a bowl, add pepper, vinegar, sugar, and salt and whisk until all the sugar dissolves. Remove the zest from the lemon oil you made in step one and add the oil to the dressing. Add onion and let it sit for 15 minutes.
4. Add cucumber, cilantro, carrot, watercress, basil, and mint to the bowl with the rice. Add dressing and toss. Serve.

▷ Stuffed peppers

Servings: 4 (32 calories per serving)

Total time: 25 minutes (plus 75 minutes of baking time)

Ingredients

- 4 bell peppers, any color
- 1 teaspoon dried oregano
- Black pepper and salt to taste
- 220 g ground beef (7.76 oz)
- 1 small onion, chopped
- 4 teaspoons olive oil
- 2 garlic cloves, chopped
- ½ teaspoon cinnamon
- 1/3 cup lentils
- ½ cup long-grain white rice
- ½ teaspoon ground cumin
- 2 tablespoon tomato paste
- ½ teaspoon, ground dill, chopped (you can also use mint or parsley)

Directions

1. Preheat the oven to 200°C. Remove the tops from the peppers and hollow them out. Sprinkle pepper and salt inside the peppers and set aside.
2. Heat a little oil in a skillet and add onions and garlic. Cook for three minutes and add oregano, cumin, cinnamon, and beef. Cook while stirring the meat until it loses its pink color. Add a tablespoon of tomato paste and stir until the meat darkens. Add lentils, rice, and broth while stirring. Remove from heat and leave standing

until the liquid gets absorbed and the mixture cools. Season with pepper and salt.

3. Divide the rice mix into the peppers and return the tops. Arrange the peppers in a baking dish. Combine the remaining oil and tomato paste with a cup of water and pour them into the baking dish with the peppers. Cover using foil and bake for 75 minutes or until the peppers become tender.

4. Transfer them carefully onto a serving plate. Put the cooking liquid in a skillet and boil until you have a thick sauce. Remove and spice with dill. Season with pepper and salt and serve alongside the stuffed peppers.

▷ **Chicken Shawarma**

Servings: 3 (314 calories per serving)

Total time: 90 minutes

Ingredients

For chicken

- ½ teaspoon black pepper
- 1 teaspoon garlic powder
- 2 tablespoons olive oil
- 3 chicken breasts, boneless, stripped
- 2 teaspoons ground cumin
- 1 teaspoon cayenne pepper

- 1 teaspoon paprika
- 1 teaspoon coriander, ground
- 1 teaspoon salt

For the wraps

- 3 small pita bread
- ¼ cup parsley, chopped
- 2 cups lettuce, chopped
- 2 cucumbers, diced
- 1 tomato, diced

For the sauce

- 1 cup Greek yogurt, plain
- ¼ teaspoon ground black pepper, ground
- 1 tablespoon Dijon mustard
- 1 tablespoon lemon juice
- ¼ teaspoon salt
- ½ teaspoon garlic

Directions

1. Mix the chicken strips with all the seasoning and a tablespoon of oil in a Ziploc bag. Remove the air and seal. Let them marinate for an hour or overnight in the fridge.
2. Preheat your oven to 200°C. Spread the chicken on a baking pan on one layer and bake for 20

minutes until crispy and well done. Remove and cool.

3. Serve in pita bread with parsley, cucumber, lettuce, and tomato.

4. Use a bowl to combine the sauce ingredients and stir till smooth. Drizzle on the shawarma while serving. If you have leftovers, store everything in the fridge in its own airtight container for up to four days. If you like, you can pre-cook the chicken and freeze it until you are ready to make the shawarma. It will last for two months.

▷ **Hawaiian tuna bowl**

Servings: 4 (435 calories per serving)

Total time: 25 minutes

Ingredients

- 1 avocado, diced
- 1 cup sushi rice
- 2 cups sushi-grade tuna
- 1 ½ cups water
- 1 teaspoon rice vinegar
- ¼ cup tamari
- 2 onions, sliced
- 1 teaspoon sesame oil
- 1 cucumber, sliced
- sesame seeds and microgreens for garnishing

Directions

1. Rinse the rice in a colander until you get clear water. Put it in a pot with the water and boil. Simmer for 20 minutes.
2. As the rice cooks, cut the tuna into chunks.
3. Mix the rice vinegar, tamari, and sesame oil in a bowl and add the tuna. Stir to coat all the pieces. Add the onion and stir some more.
4. When the rice is done, serve. Top it with the tuna, cucumber, and some avocado. Garnish with the sesame seeds and microgreens.

▷ Vegetable rice and edamame

Servings: 1 (394 calories per serving)

Total time: 5 minutes

Ingredients

- ½ cup cooked brown rice
- 1 cup roasted vegetables
- ¼ avocado, diced
- ¼ cup edamame
- 2 tablespoons cilantro, chopped
- 2 tablespoons scallions, chopped
- 2 tablespoons lime vinaigrette

Directions

1. Arrange the edamame, vegetables, rice, and avocado in a bowl.
2. Top with cilantro and scallions. Drizzle the vinaigrette and serve.

▷ Vegetable sandwich

Servings: 4 (389 calories per serving)

Total time: 30 minutes

Ingredients

- ½ avocado
- 1 red bell pepper, cut into pieces
- 70g provolone, sliced
- 2 tablespoons white wine vinegar
- 1/3 cup pepperoncini, sliced
- 1 tablespoon oregano, chopped
- ½ cup cucumber, sliced
- 1 tablespoon Greek yogurt
- 2 garlic cloves, minced
- 1 cup arugula
- 12 slices whole-wheat bread
- ½ cup red onion, sliced
- 1/3 cup tomatoes
- 70g mozzarella cheese, sliced

Directions

1. Empty the avocado into a bowl and use a fork to mash it. Add yogurt, vinegar, garlic, and oregano, and keep mashing until smooth. Spread the mixture on the bread slices.
2. Top four slices with arugula, mozzarella, tomatoes, and onions. Place the other four on top and top with cucumbers, provolone, peppers, and pepperoncini. Place the rest of the slices on top.
3. Use bamboo picks to help you cut the sandwiches into halves and serve.

▷ Chicken salad with dressing

Servings: 4 (234 calories per serving)

Total time: 5 minutes

Ingredients

For the salad

- 1 head lettuce, chopped
- 1 cucumber, sliced
- 1 cup purple cabbage, chopped
- 3 radishes, sliced
- 1 cup tomatoes, halved
- 1 carrot, shredded
- ¼ red onion, sliced
- 1 chicken breast, cooked and sliced

- ½ cup croutons, seasoned

For the dressing

- 2 tablespoons whole milk
- 1/8 teaspoon onion powder
- 1 teaspoon lemon juice
- 1 tablespoon mayonnaise
- ¼ cup sour cream
- ½ tablespoon parsley
- salt and pepper to taste
- ½ teaspoon dill
- 1/8 teaspoon garlic powder

Directions

1. Place the cabbage, tomatoes, lettuce, cucumber, carrot, red onion, radishes, and chicken breast on a serving plate. Pour the dressing and combine. Top with croutons to serve.
2. To make the dressing, mix the ingredients and whisk until smooth.
3. Season the sides with pepper and salt if you start with raw chicken breast. Heat oil in a skillet and cook the chicken for seven minutes per side until it is well done. Let it cool before slicing.
4. You can also make the salad ahead of time. Prep the vegetables and store them in a container. Store the dressing in a different container and

combine when ready to serve. This salad is best eaten fresh, but leftovers can be refrigerated for three days in an airtight container. Do not refrigerate the croutons though. They get mushy.

▷ **Shrimp toast**

Servings: 8 (400 calories per serving)

Total time: 45 minutes

Ingredients

- ¼ cup heavy cream
- 1/8 teaspoon white pepper
- ½ teaspoon salt
- 8 slices white bread
- ½ cup vegetable oil
- 1 large egg and 1 egg white
- 1 cup raw shrimp
- 2 tablespoons green onions
- 85 gm (approx 3 oz) cream cheese
- 1 teaspoon garlic, minced
- 2 tablespoons parsley, minced

Directions

1. Mix the egg white, egg, parsley, salt, white pepper, green onions, shrimp, and garlic in a blender and blend until you have a chunky mix.

Add the cheese and pulse to smoothness. Add heavy cream and pulse for another minute without over-processing.

2. Spread ¼ cup of the shrimp mixture onto a bread slice.

3. Heat oil in a skillet and toast the bread in batches. Fry the shrimp side for three minutes and turn. Fry the other side for a minute and drain on a paper towel.

4. Cut the toast into quarters to serve and drizzle with a sauce of choice if desired, or eat plain.

▷ **Mandarin chicken salad**

Servings: 4 (314 calories per serving)

Total time: 55 minutes

Ingredients

For the chicken

- 2 boneless chicken breasts
- ¼ cup almonds
- 5 cups spinach
- 2 green onions, chopped
- 4 mandarins, separated and peeled
- 1 cucumber, sliced
- sesame seeds
- 1 avocado, diced

For the vinaigrette

- 1/3 cup olive oil
- 1 teaspoon Dijon mustard
- ¼ cup lemon juice
- pepper and salt to taste
- ½ teaspoon honey
- 1 garlic clove, minced

Directions

1. To make the vinaigrette, mix all the ingredients and whisk. Store in the fridge.
2. When making the chicken, mix some of the vinaigrette with the chicken, and let it marinate for about 30 minutes.
3. Preheat the oven to 220°C. Bake the chicken for 25 minutes.
4. Shred the chicken with a fork and mix with the rest of the ingredients. Drizzle the rest of the vinaigrette and serve.

▷ Shrimp salad

Servings: 4 (251 calories per serving)

Total time: 25 minutes

Ingredients

For shrimp

- 20 pieces prepared shrimp
- 1 tablespoon olive oil
- 1 tablespoon lemon juice
- 2 tablespoons garlic, minced
- 1 teaspoon paprika
- ½ teaspoon black pepper
- 1 teaspoon salt
- ½ tablespoon Italian seasoning

For salad

- 6 cups mixed greens
- ¼ teaspoon black pepper
- 1 tablespoon olive oil
- 1 tablespoon lemon juice
- 1 avocado, sliced
- 1 red bell pepper, sliced
- ½ red onion, sliced
- ¼ teaspoon salt

Directions

1. Mix the shrimp, seasoning, garlic, pepper, oil, paprika, and salt in a bowl and toss to coat the shrimp. Marinate for 20 minutes.

2. Use bamboo skewers to thread the shrimp.

3. Brush oil on a grill pan and preheat it for three minutes. Put the skewers on the grill and cook for four minutes per side until the shrimp becomes opaque.

4. Mix the salad ingredients in a bowl. Unthread the shrimp into the salad.

5. Mix pepper, salt, lemon juice, and olive oil in a different bowl. Pour the dressing on the salad and mix.

▷ **Chopped Cobb and chicken**

Servings: 1 (410 calories)

Total time: 5 minutes

Ingredients

- 2 cups lettuce
- 2 tablespoons blue cheese dressing
- ¼ cup tomato, chopped
- ¼ cup cucumber, chopped
- ½ egg, boiled and chopped
- 1 chicken breast, roasted and stripped
- ¼ cup mushrooms, sliced
- ¼ cannellini beans

Directions

1. Put the lettuce in a bowl and add a tablespoon of the dressing to coat.
2. Arrange the rest of the ingredients in rows on the lettuce.
3. Drizzle the rest of the dressing and serve.

▷ Vegetable wrap and hummus

Servings: 4 (320 calories per serving)

Total time: 23 minutes

Ingredients

- 2 zucchini, sliced
- 2 teaspoons olive oil
- 1 red bell pepper, sliced
- black pepper and salt to taste
- 1 cup hummus
- ¼ cup mint leaves
- ¼ cup pine nuts
- ¼ cup spinach
- ½ cup red onion, sliced
- 4 pieces whole wheat bread

Directions

1. Preheat a pan. Brush the zucchini with oil and sprinkle pepper and salt. Grill for four minutes per side.
2. Spread a quarter of the hummus on each slice of bread. Sprinkle pine nuts and top with zucchini, bell pepper, spinach, onions, and mint. Roll up the bread and cut it in half. Serve.

▷ Chicken rolls

Servings: 6 (243 calories per serving)

Total time: 20 minutes

Ingredients

For rolls

- 1 cup rice noodles
- 6 rice wrappers
- 1 cup cooked chicken breast
- 1 cucumber
- 1 carrot
- ¼ cup cilantro, chopped

For dipping sauce

- Black bean sauce
- 1 tablespoon water

- 1 tablespoon peanut butter
- ½ tablespoon honey
- ½ tablespoon lime juice
- 1 tablespoon peanuts, roasted and chopped

Directions

1. Follow the package instructions to make the noodles and dry them out.
2. Fill a bowl with warm water and dip the rice wrappers one at a time for a second.
3. Place some carrots and cucumbers on the wrapper and roll. Leave two inches on each side. Top with the noodles, cilantro, and chicken.
4. Roll the wrapper from the bottom. Fold the sides inward as you roll to seal the mixture in the roll.
5. To make the sauce, mix all the ingredients and stir them to make a uniform and smooth mixture. Sprinkle with roasted peanuts.

In chapter nine, you will find a complete list of recipes you can use to make your dinners enjoyable and healthy.

Chapter 9
The Recipes - Dinner

In January 2019, on a slow Saturday evening, Jennifer went out with her friends for dinner. That night, she hit rock bottom, eating a kilo of carrot cake and a pile of seafood. Before dinner, her suit didn't quite fit. After the crazy meal, it was not a surprise the suit didn't fit at all. She felt horrible – both emotionally and physically. Her health was terrible, and she knew it. She decided to change things. Jennifer had tried losing weight in 2016 but without much success. She was a chubby kid and an even chubbier adult, weighing 275 pounds. Once she had managed to come down to 220 pounds but put the weight back on.

Jennifer had to come to terms with one truth – weight management is 90 percent what you eat. She tried many diets, but anxiety, social pressures, boredom, and stress would cause her to eat back all the weight she lost. In

2019, at 43, she started learning about nutrition. She learned terms like glycogen, sugar, insulin, carbohydrates, ketosis, etc. In the process, she learned about intermittent fasting. It seemed crazy because she could not imagine going more than five hours without food. After fighting the concept, she decided to give it a chance.

In two months, she lost 55 pounds. Jennifer was losing weight every week. Her body fat went to 16.2%, from 26.5%. Even though she would occasionally hit plateaus, three more months later, Jennifer had lost another 75 pounds. She kept trusting the process. She felt lighter, more in control of her body, and healthier. Now she could go sixteen hours without food. It was not too hard. She even tried the one meal a day method and took up weightlifting to build muscles.

As her life changed around this eating method, she had to admit to another truth – she was addicted to sugar. She struggled with that addiction, falling off the wagon more times than she cared to admit. Jennifer learned that she could grow and overcome the false beliefs she had embraced around food. She finally stood against the bombardment of processed foods we face today and prevailed. She removed sugar substitutes from her diet and moderated her intake. She learned that what you eat at any time of the day is vital to good health.

For Jennifer, IF is not just about refraining from food for a period, even though it is an integral part. It is about the changes it forces you to make to your life. It is about learning commitment to self, resilience, and trusting the process. It is about choosing the right food for you. Here, you will find a list of recipes to help you make a similar journey to Jennifer's when preparing your dinners.

▷ Turkey tacos

Servings: 4 (472 calories per serving)

Total time: 30 minutes

Ingredients

- 2 teaspoons vegetable oil
- 1 garlic clove, minced
- 1 red onion, chopped
- 1 pound lean turkey
- 8 whole-grain tortillas
- 1 avocado, sliced
- 1 tablespoon taco seasoning
- ¼ cup sour cream
- 1 cup lettuce, chopped
- ½ cup Mexican cheese

Directions

1. Heat oil in a pan and cook the onion for five minutes. Add garlic and cook for another minute.

2. Add turkey and let it cook until it browns. It should take about five minutes. Season and add a cup of water. Simmer for seven minutes.

3. Once the turkey is cooked, divide it between the tortillas and top with cheese, lettuce, sour cream, and avocado. Serve.

▷ Noodles served with salmon

Servings: 4 (516 calories per serving)

Total time: 40 minutes

Ingredients

- 1/2 cup peanut oil
- 3 shallots, sliced
- 1 tablespoon ginger, chopped
- 1 lemongrass stalk, grated
- 80g (2.82 oz) chili paste
- 2 tablespoons olive oil
- 1 ½ tablespoon honey
- 600g (1 ½ pounds) salmon filet
- 2 ½ teaspoon caster sugar
- 240g (8.46 oz) noodles
- 1/3 cup lime juice
- 2 teaspoons fish sauce
- ½ teaspoon chili flakes
- sesame seeds

Directions

1. Preheat the oven to 220°C. Heat the peanut oil in a saucepan for a minute. Add the shallot, lemongrass, ginger, and salt. Cook while stirring for six minutes. Cool.
2. Mix the chili paste, honey, and olive oil in a bowl. Place the salmon on a baking tray. Rub the honey mix on the salmon and season with salt. Roast in the oven for 15 minutes. Let it rest for five minutes.
3. Prepare the noodles as per the instructions on the packet and drain.
4. Mix fish sauce, chili flakes, lime juice, and sugar with the shallot oil mix. Put the noodles in a bowl with most of the shallot oil and mix. Arrange on a plate and flake the salmon onto the plate. Drizzle the rest of the shallot oil with sesame seeds and serve at room temperature or chill it.

▷ Steak served with toasted sweet potatoes

Servings: 2 (90 calories per serving)

Total time: 30 minutes

Ingredients

- 2 sweet potatoes
- 2 tablespoon olive oil

- black pepper and salt
- 1/3 cup watercress
- 1/3 cup red bell peppers, sliced
- 4 ounces sirloin, cooked and sliced
- hot sauce to serve

Directions

1. Preheat the oven to 200°C preheat.
2. Slice the sweet potatoes into long rectangular shapes.
3. Coat the sweet potatoes with one tablespoon of oil and some salt and pepper to taste. Arrange them on a baking tray and cook them until they are tender and slightly browned. This should take 15 minutes.
4. Serve the sweet potatoes on two plates and divide the bell peppers between them. Top with steak. Use a bowl to combine the watercress, the remaining olive oil, and the sauce, then drizzle them on the steak. Season with black pepper and serve.

▷ Cajun fried cabbage with chicken sausages

Servings: 2 (300 calories per serving)

Total time: 35 minutes

Ingredients

- 2 tablespoons canola oil
- 4 pieces chicken sausages, sliced into pieces
- 1 yellow onion, sliced
- Salt
- 1 tablespoon unsalted butter
- ¼ red pepper
- 1 head green cabbage, cored and sliced
- 2 garlic cloves, minced
- 3 tablespoons apple cider vinegar
- ½ apple, cored and sliced
- 1 scallion, sliced
- Hot sauce – to serve

Directions

1. Place a skillet on medium heat for a minute. Add oil and the sausage slices in one layer. Let them cook for two minutes until they turn brown. Flip and brown the other side. Remove and set aside.
2. Add onion and salt and sprinkle a little water in the pan. Cook while scraping any sausage bits stuck at the bottom of the pan. When the onions are tender and slightly brown, add the pepper, cabbage, and a little more salt and cook for eight minutes. If at some point the pan seems dry, add a little water.

3. Add the vinegar and garlic and cook until most of the vinegar evaporates. Keep stirring. Add butter and let it melt, then add the sausage and apple. Let them cook until the apples become tender.

4. Sprinkle the scallion and serve with the hot sauce.

▷ Lemon flavored chicken

Servings: 2 (456 calories per serving)

Total time: 10 minutes

Ingredients

- 1 teaspoon corn flour
- 1 teaspoon soy sauce
- 4 spring onions, sliced
- lemon juice and zest from 1 lemon
- 150g (1/2 pound) chicken breast filet, sliced
- 2 teaspoons coconut oil
- 1 capsicum, sliced
- 1 cup chicken stock
- 1 broccoli, cut into florets
- 1 carrot, sliced

Directions

1. Mix the lemon juice, soy sauce, and corn flour.
2. Pour the oil into a skillet and heat it. Add chicken, broccoli, carrot, and capsicum and stir. Cook for three minutes.
3. Pour the soy and lemon mix into the pan and add the onions and chicken stock. Bring to boil and then simmer for two minutes on low heat. When the sauce becomes thick, the chicken is ready.
4. Sprinkle the lemon zest and serve on its own or with rice.

▷ Chicken burgers

Servings: 4 (435 calories per serving)

Total time: 20 minutes

Ingredients

For the burgers

- 2 teaspoons olive oil
- 1 teaspoon cinnamon
- 1 onion, chopped
- ¼ cup yogurt, plain
- 1 teaspoon coriander
- ¼ teaspoon red pepper flakes
- ¼ cup parsley, chopped
- 1 ½ teaspoons salt

- 1 pound lean chicken
- 3 tablespoons pomegranate molasses
- 2 garlic cloves, minced

For the fixings

- 1 red onion, sliced
- 4 wheat buns, toasted
- 1 cucumber, sliced
- 1 tomato, sliced
- 1 lettuce head

Directions

1. Heat olive oil in a pan. Add coriander, onion, cinnamon, ½ teaspoon salt, pepper flakes, and season with pepper. Cook till tender. Add parsley and garlic and cook for a minute more.
2. Transfer to a bowl and let cool.
3. Add the chicken and yogurt and mix evenly. Season with the rest of the salt and shape into patties.
4. Cook the patties in a skillet for five minutes per side until they brown. Brush the burgers with molasses and let them rest for five minutes. Assemble the burgers and serve.

▷ Vegetables served with Salmon

Servings: 4 (281 calories per serving)

Total time: 25 minutes

Ingredients

- 1 zucchini, halved
- 2 red bell peppers, halved
- 1 red onion, cut into wedges
- 1 tablespoon olive oil
- pepper and salt to taste
- 1 ¼ pounds salmon filet pounds, cut into portions
- 1 lemon, cut into wedges
- ¼ cup basil

Directions

1. Set up and preheat the grill.
2. Brush the peppers, onion, and zucchini with oil and sprinkle with salt. Season the salmon with pepper and salt as well.
3. Put the salmon pieces and vegetables on the grill and cook. Turn the vegetables occasionally and remove them once tender. It should take about six minutes for the vegetables to cook. Cook the salmon for ten minutes without turning it.

4. Once the salmon and vegetables are cool, chop the vegetables and put them in a bowl. Serve the fish with the vegetables and garnish with basil and a lemon wedge.

▷ Scampi shrimp served with pasta

Servings: 6 (511 calories per serving)

Total time: 40 minutes

Ingredients

- 1 packet pasta
- 4 tablespoon butter
- 2 shallots, diced
- 2 tablespoon olive oil
- 2 garlic cloves, minced
- Pepper and salt to taste
- Red pepper flakes to taste
- 1 pound shrimp, deveined and peeled
- ½ cup dry white wine
- 2 tablespoons butter
- 1 lemon
- ¼ cup parsley, chopped

Directions

1. Cook the pasta and drain it.
2. Melt half of the butter and mix it with olive oil in a large pan. Cook the garlic, shallots, and red pepper flakes for three minutes. Season the shrimp with pepper and salt and add them to the pan. Cook for three more minutes and remove.
3. Juice the lemon and pour the juice into the skillet with the wine. Boil, and be sure to scrape the food bits at the bottom of the skillet. Melt the rest of the butter in the skillet and simmer. Add the shrimp and pasta and toss. Top with parsley and remove from heat.
4. Season with pepper and salt, and serve with a sprinkle of olive oil.

▷ Spaghetti Bolognese

Servings: 4 (450 calories per serving)

Total time: 90 minutes

Ingredients

- 3 tablespoons olive oil
- 1 spaghetti squash
- ½ teaspoon garlic powder
- Pepper and salt to taste
- 1 onion, chopped

- 1 ¼ pounds ground turkey
- 2 garlic cloves, chopped
- Basil
- ¼ cup cremini mushrooms, sliced
- 3 cups tomatoes, diced
- 2 tablespoons tomato sauce

Directions

1. Preheat oven to 200°C. Halve the spaghetti squash and deseed. Rub the halves with half the oil and season with pepper, salt, and garlic powder. Put the squashes on a baking sheet with the skin facing up and roast for 35 minutes. Let cool.

2. As they roast, heat the remaining oil in a pan and fry the onions seasoned with pepper and salt. Throw in the turkey and cook until browned. It will take seven minutes. Add the garlic and cook for a minute more.

3. Move the turkey to the side of the pan and put the mushrooms on the other side. Cook for five minutes, and then mix the mushrooms and the turkey. Add tomato sauce and the tomatoes and let them simmer for ten minutes.

4. As the sauce simmers, remove the squash and plate. Spoon the turkey mix on the squash and sprinkle with basil to serve.

▷ **Mushroom stroganoff**

Servings: 2 (251 calories per serving)

Total time: 20 minutes

Ingredients

- 1 cup mushrooms, trimmed and sliced
- 1 pickled onion, sliced
- 1 red onion, chopped
- 2 cornichons, sliced
- 2 garlic cloves, minced
- 1 tablespoon baby capers
- Paprika to taste
- olive oil as required
- 4 sprigs parsley, chopped
- 5 ml whisky
- ½ cup sour cream

Directions

1. Heat a pan and dry fry the red onions and mushrooms for five minutes. Shake them to make one layer, and keep stirring as you cook them.
2. Drizzle a tablespoon of oil and add the pickled onions, parsley, capers, and garlic. Cook for three minutes, then tilt the pan to add the whisky. It will light up. When the flames die down, add paprika, sour cream, and parsley, and mix.

3. If the mixture is too thick, add a tablespoon of boiling water. Season with pepper and salt to taste. Serve with rice.

▷ Southern rice and pork

Servings: 4 (512 calories per serving)

Total time: 45 minutes

Ingredients

- 1/3 cup peanut oil
- 4 cups long-grain rice
- ½ cup chili bean sauce
- 4 garlic cloves, sliced
- ½ cup pork, minced
- 1 bunch chives
- Fried egg – for serving

Directions

1. Cook the garlic in a pan until it turns brown. Remove and set aside.
2. Put the pork in the oil and cook for seven minutes until it is slightly browned. Add the sauce and cook for two more minutes.
3. Add rice and chives and cook for three minutes. Top with fried egg and garlic to serve.

▷ Cauliflower rice and chicken

Servings: 4 (427 calories per serving)

Total time: 35 minutes

Ingredients

- 2 tablespoon grapeseed oil
- 2 teaspoon rice vinegar
- 1 boneless chicken breast
- 4 eggs
- 2 tablespoon soy sauce
- 2 red bell peppers, chopped
- 1 onion, chopped
- 2 carrots, chopped
- ½ cup peas
- 2 garlic cloves, chopped
- 4 scallions, chopped
- pepper and salt to taste
- 4 cups cauliflower rice

Directions

1. Cook the chicken in a hot skillet for four minutes per side. Let it rest on a chopping board before slicing it. As you wait for it to cool, scramble the eggs for two minutes and put them in a bowl.
2. Add the carrots, onions, and bell peppers to the skillet and cook for five minutes, stir the garlic in

and cook for another minute. Finally, toss the peas and scallions.

3. Add soy sauce, cauliflower, pepper, salt, and rice vinegar, and mix. Let the mixture sit for three minutes without stirring. Add the chicken and eggs. Serve warm.

▷ Ginger rice and chicken

Servings: 4 (510 calories per serving)

Total time: 35 minutes

Ingredients

- 1 cup all-purpose flour
- 2 scallions, sliced
- 2 eggs, beaten
- 1 cup breadcrumbs
- 3 cups cooked white rice
- 4 chicken cutlets
- pepper and salt
- vegetable oil as required
- 3 garlic cloves, minced
- 2 teaspoons ginger, minced
- 3 heads bok choy, chopped
- katsu sauce – to serve

Directions

1. Divide the eggs, breadcrumbs, and flour into three bowls. Season the cutlets and dip them in the egg. Remove excess eggs and dip them in the breadcrumbs to coat them evenly. Finally, dip them in the flour and plate them.
2. Heat some of the oil in a pan and cook the chicken for four minutes until brown and crispy. Turn the chicken and cook the other side for four minutes as well. Remove and set aside to drain.
3. Heat two tablespoons of oil in another skillet and add ginger and garlic. Cook for 30 seconds. Add bok choy and salt and stir for a minute. Add the rice and cook until it warms through. This should take two minutes. Finally, add the scallions and season.
4. Serve the rice and chicken with katsu sauce.

▷ Beef stir-fry

Servings: 4 (450 calories per serving)

Total time: 30 minutes

Ingredients

- 1 ½ pounds steak, cut into four pieces
- pepper and salt
- ¼ cup soy sauce

- 1 chili pepper, chopped
- 2 tablespoons olive oil
- 2 teaspoons sugar
- 1 bunch scallions, sliced
- 2 tablespoons lime juice
- 2 garlic cloves, grated
- ½ cups mushrooms, sliced
- ½ cup baby corn
- ¼ cup peas
- 1 red bell pepper, sliced

Directions

1. Mix the chili pepper, lime juice, sugar, and soy sauce in a bowl and whisk until all the sugar dissolves. Season the beef and coat it in the soy sauce mixture.
2. Heat oil in a skillet and add the steak. Cook while stirring for five minutes. Remove it and set aside.
3. Let some of the liquid in the pan evaporate so that you have a thick sauce. Add scallions and garlic, and cook for a minute. Add mushrooms and cook for three minutes before adding the bell pepper, snow peas, and baby corn. Cook until the vegetables become tender. Return the steak and mix. Cook for a minute and remove. Serve hot.

▷ **Pad Thai with basil**

Servings: 2 (593 calories per serving)

Total time: 30 minutes

Ingredients

- ½ cup rice noodles
- 1 handful peanuts
- sesame oil as needed
- 2 garlic cloves, minced
- 1/8 cup tofu
- 3 tablespoons soy sauce
- 3 teaspoons tamarind paste
- 1 shallot, sliced
- 2 teaspoons chili sauce
- 2 limes
- ¼ beansprouts
- 1 cup broccoli (you can also use asparagus or baby corn)
- 2 eggs
- chili flakes – as needed
- 2 tablespoons olive oil
- 1 small head lettuce
- basil

Directions

1. Prepare the noodles and drain them under running water. Sprinkle with sesame oil.
2. Toast peanuts in a pan on medium heat for five minutes and grind till fine. Set them aside in a bowl. Prepare the garlic and mix it with the tofu to make a paste. Add one teaspoon of sesame oil, tamarind paste, chili sauce, and a teaspoon of soy. Squeeze in half of the lime.
3. Fry the shallot over high heat with a bit of sesame oil. Add the broccoli and fry for four minutes.
4. Add beansprouts, noodles, and a little water if it feels too dry. Toss and heat for a minute.
5. Wipe the pan and fry the eggs with olive oil. Season with chili flakes. As you wait, trim the lettuce and prepare for serving.
6. Mix the egg with the herbs and sprinkle the nuts. Serve with the remaining lime.

In the final chapter of this book, I will provide you with some easy exercises that you can pair with intermittent fasting to speed up your weight loss and keep you healthy.

Chapter 10
The 7-Day Exercise Routine

C hapter 4 debunks the myth that you should not exercise while fasting. On the contrary, it is actually recommended to combine IF with exercise. Losing weight and gaining muscle is more than exercise and calories. It is about hormone optimization. Combining exercise and IF achieves that. Your growth hormone levels increase, and you become more insulin sensitive, which keeps you youthful and lean. It is recommended to exercise in the morning before you break your fast so that you support the natural circadian rhythm. In addition, time your workout so that you do not eat immediately after exercise to make the most out of hormone optimization.

Research shows that waiting about two hours after exercising before eating increases the growth hormone and helps you burn more fat. If your schedule is too packed to exercise in the morning, exercise when you can, but do not eat immediately after a workout. Do any exercise you enjoy. Doing cardio during fasting may be difficult initially, though, as your body adapts to using fat as a fuel source. Avoid overextending yourself within the first two weeks. If it proves too difficult, begin with high-intensity training and introduce cardio slowly.

Some people opt to combine IF and weight lifting. If you go down that road, be aware of the role glucose plays in repairing muscle repair after a session. When you weight lift while fasting, the body has already depleted your glycogen stores. You should, therefore, prioritize a meal immediately after your workout. Unlike cardio or HIIT, weight lifting stresses your body enough to need energy immediately afterward. If possible, the ideal time to do your weight lifting is after eating.

To put it in simple terms, it is not only okay to exercise while fasting; it is very beneficial. You can do weight training and cardio during the fasted state or after you have broken your fast. I will provide a list of exercises and a seven-day plan to start with. Feel free to tweak this program to make it your own and accommodate your needs. Like with other IF-related things, do not be afraid to experiment with how you organize your workout to find what works for you.

▷ Lunges

Lunges target the lower body. To perform a lunge, begin in an upright position, with feet slightly apart and arms at your waist. Step forward with the left foot and bend your knees. Stop when the left thigh is parallel to the ground. Do not let it extend beyond the left foot. Push off your left foot and return to the neutral position. Repeat with the right leg. This is one rep.

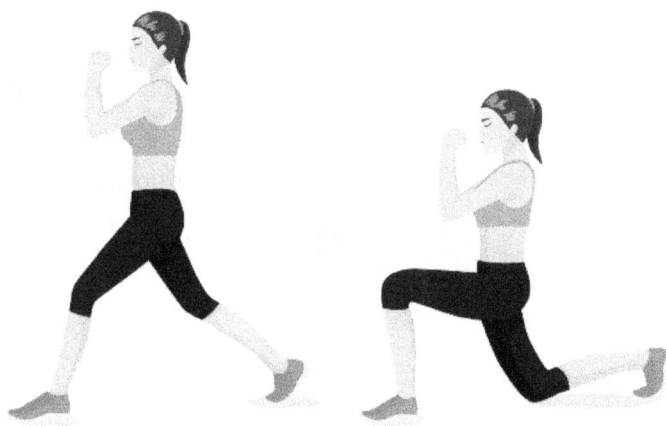

▷ **Walking lunges**

By performing the lunge while moving instead of being stationary, you introduce aspects of balance, mobility, and stability. Start by doing the stationary lunge described above, but instead of returning to the neutral position, after standing up, step forward with the right foot and repeat the movement.

▷ Wall pushups

The pushup is an effective bodyweight movement you can do daily. This exercise targets the back, shoulders, chest, and arms and builds up your strength as you increase the number of reps. The wall pushup is a variation of the regular pushup and is suitable for beginners. Stand in front of a wall, an arm's length away from it. Keep your feet slightly apart. Hold the wall with both arms at shoulder level and width, with fingers pointing upwards. Bend your elbows slowly and start leaning toward the wall. Push yourself close to the wall while keeping your back straight. Then, push back slowly to your starting position.

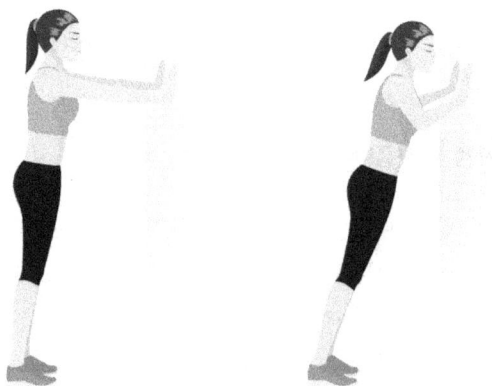

▷ Squats

Squats are an excellent exercise to work out your lower body, boost flexibility, and increase your core strength because they engage many muscle groups. To do a squat, start straight with feet slightly apart and arms to the sides. Tighten your core and lift your chin and chest. Next, push yourself back, hinging at the hips, and bend your knees as if sitting down. Keep dropping until your thighs are parallel to the ground without bending the knees outward or inward. Pause for a breath and then return to the neutral position. That is one rep.

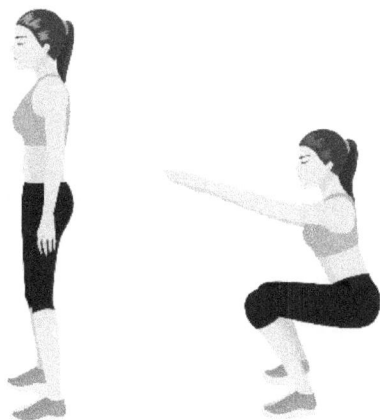

▷ **Burpees**

Burpees are effective as a whole-body exercise that builds endurance and strength. To do a burpee, stand tall with feet apart and arms at your sides. Start to squat while extending your hands in front. When your hands reach the ground, straighten your legs so that you are in a pushup position. Jump to your feet by bending the waist and standing up, bringing your hands over your head. Jump. That makes one rep.

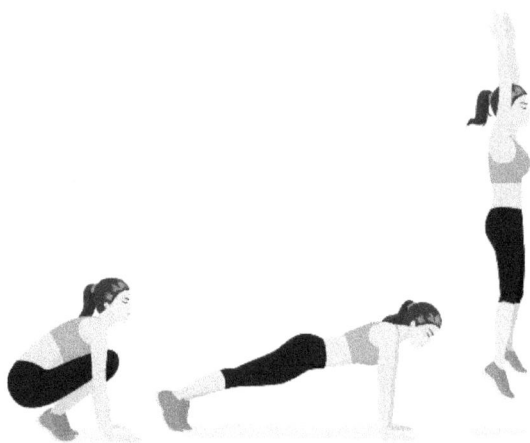

▷ Side planks

If your body is going to be healthy, it needs a strong core. The side plank and the plank strengthen your core. It is all about the muscle-mind connection and controlling your movements. To perform the side plank, lie on the left side and stack your feet. Next, lift your upper body with your left forearm, ensuring the elbow is under the shoulder. Tighten your core and lift your knees and hips from the ground. Ensure that your head is in line with your spine. Hold for two seconds and return slowly to the starting position. Repeat for the desired counts and then switch sides.

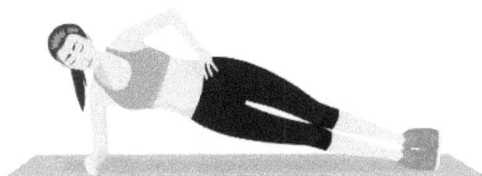

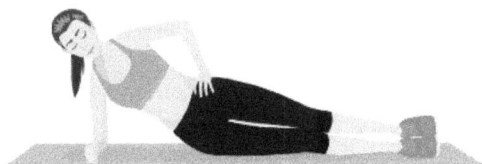

▷ **Planks**

The standard plank targets your core. It stabilizes it without putting a strain on your back. To execute the movement, get in the pushup position and plant your toes and hands on the ground. Straighten your back and tighten your core. Tuck your chin. Maintain the tension throughout your body and engage your abs, glutes, shoulders, triceps, and quads. Hold for 30 seconds to make one rep.

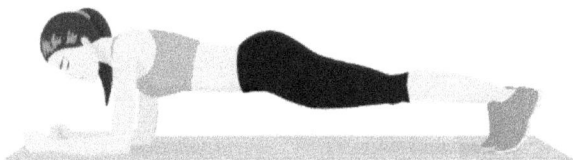

▷ **The bridge**

The bridge works your glutes and is the perfect exercise to give you *a* tight bottom. Begin the movement by lying flat on your back and facing up. Bend your knees with your palms down and arms to the side. Raise your hips from your heels and squeeze your hamstrings, glutes, and core. Keep your shoulders and upper back on the ground. Pause for a second and relax. This completes one rep.

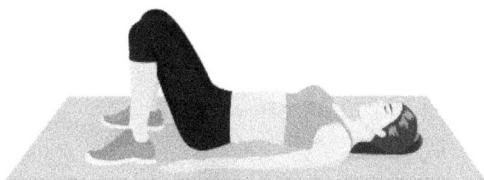

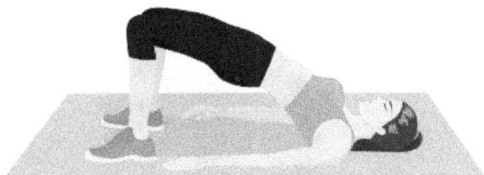

▷ **The donkey kick**

Like the bridge, this movement targets the glutes. Start on all fours. Keep your hips square on the ground and your hands directly below your shoulder. Straighten your back and push your left foot out behind you with a straight leg. Keep it flexed all through the movement. Be careful not to tilt your hips. When your foot gets to the top, tighten your glutes and go back to starting position. Repeat with the right leg to make a rep.

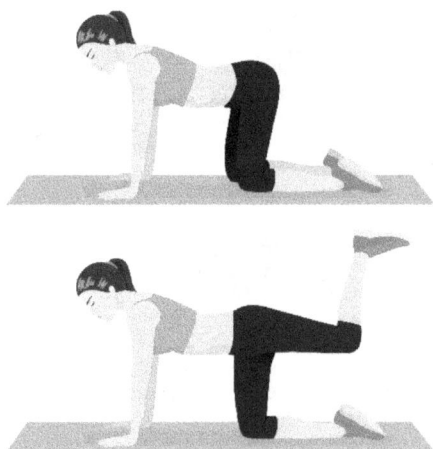

▷ **The bird dog**

This movement builds your stability and balance. You can scale it as you become better at it. To perform it, begin on all fours as if you are about to do the donkey kick. Keep the neck in a neutral position and simultaneously extend your left leg and right arm. Pause for a breath and return to neutral. Repeat with the right leg and left arm to make one rep.

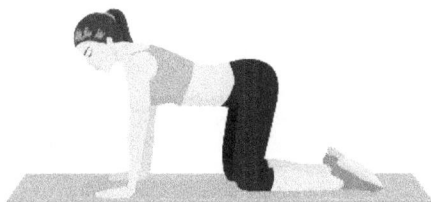

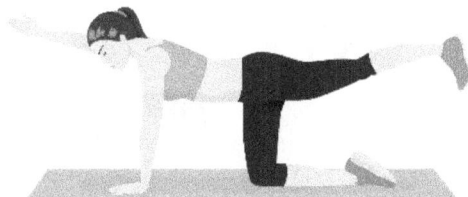

▷ **The bicycle crunch**

The bicycle crunch will mainly work your abs. Begin by lying on your back and raising your legs with bent knees. Bend the elbows and hold your neck behind the head. Bring your right elbow close to the left knee as if you were riding a bicycle and straighten them. Keep your core engaged as you perform the movement. Repeat with the left elbow and right knee to make one rep.

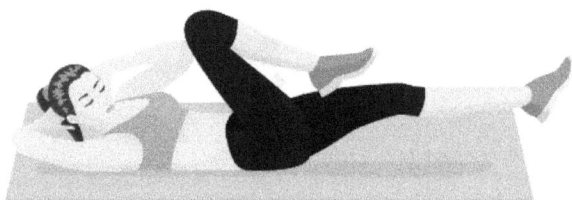

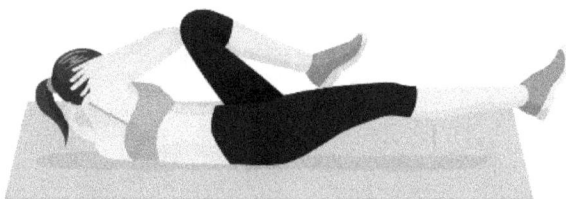

▷ **Superman**

The superman exercises your lower back. Make sure you perform it slowly to make the most out of the movement. Lie flat on your stomach and keep a neutral neck. Engage your back and core, and raise your legs and arms simultaneously. Pause at your highest point for a second before relaxing to make a single rep.

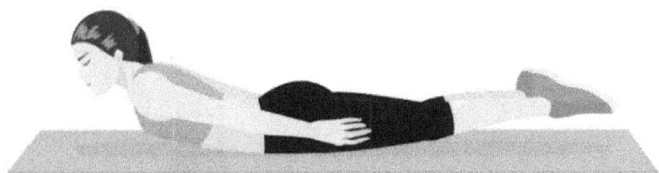

▷ Jumping jacks

The jumping jack is a good at-home cardio exercise. First, stand straight with arms at the sides. Then, jump as you open your feet as wide as possible and raise your arms above your head to almost touch. In the next jump, lower your arms and bring the legs together. That is one rep.

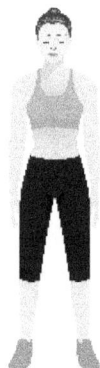

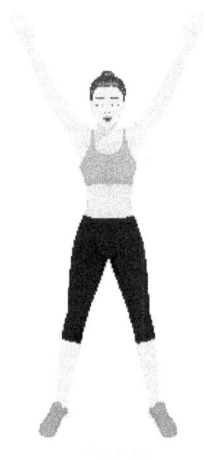

▷ The high knee

The high knee is excellent for targeting belly fat, the hips, and the inner thighs. As a beginner, do it slowly and add movements as you grow in strength and endurance. Ensure that your shoes are comfortable for this one. Stand with your feet slightly apart and arms to the side. Look ahead, engage your core and open your chest. Bring the left knee toward your chest above your waist. As you do that, move the right hand up as if you are pumping. Lower both quickly and repeat the movement with the right knee and left arm. That makes one rep.

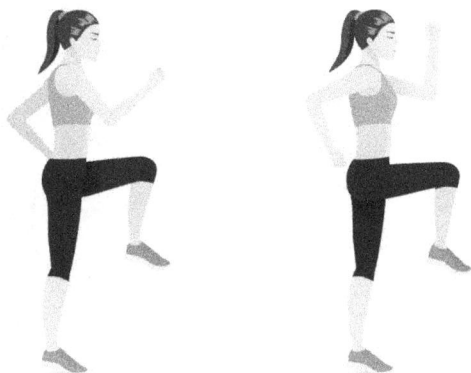

▷ **The jump rope**

The jump rope is excellent for days you want to put in some cardio without running. Ten minutes spent skipping is the equivalent of jogging for 30 minutes. When positioning your hands for the jump rope, focus on symmetry. Both hands should be about the same distance from the center of your body. Keep a minimal shoulder and elbow movement and do most of the work at the wrist. Bend your knees slightly so that you land softly after every jump. Keep your feet close to each other during a jump, and keep your spine neutral.

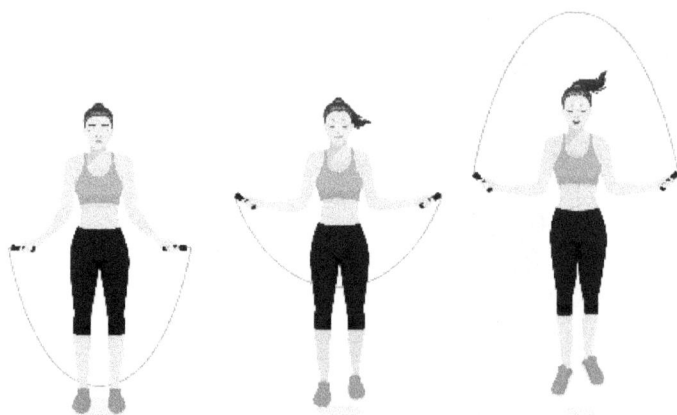

The exercise routine

You can use the following exercise routine to get started. Make sure you spend the first five minutes of your exercise warming up or stretching.

Day 1: Full body workout

- Warm-up: Jump rope (five minutes)
- Exercise 1: Squats (two sets of ten reps each)
- Exercise 2: Lunges (two sets of ten reps each)
- Rest for two minutes
- Exercise 3: Wall pushups (two sets of eight reps each)
- Exercise 4: Planks (hold for thirty seconds per rep, do three reps)
- Rest for two minutes
- Exercise 5: The bridge (two sets of seven reps each)
- Exercise 6: The bicycle crunch (two sets of seven reps each)

Day 2: Lower body workout

- Warm-up: Jumping jacks (five minutes)
- Exercise 1: Walking lunges (two sets of ten reps each)
- Exercise 2: Lunges (two sets of ten reps each)
- Rest for two minutes
- Exercise 3: Squats (three sets of five reps each)
- Exercise 4: The bridge (three sets of ten reps each)
- Rest for two minutes
- Exercise 5: The high knee (two sets of ten reps each)
- Exercise 6: The donkey kick (two sets of five reps each)

Day 3: Upper body workout

- Warm-up: Jump rope (five minutes)
- Exercise 1: Wall pushups (three sets of ten reps each)
- Exercise 2: The superman (three sets of ten reps each)
- Rest for two minutes
- Exercise 3: Planks (hold for thirty seconds per rep, do four reps)
- Exercise 4: Side planks (three sets of five reps each
- Rest for two minutes

- Exercise 5: Bicycle crunch (two sets of eight reps each)
- Exercise 6: Wall pushups (two sets of five reps each)

Day 4: Cardio workout

- Warm-up: Jump rope (five minutes)
- Exercise 1: Jumping jacks (three sets of ten reps each)
- Exercise 2: High knees (three sets of ten reps each
- Rest for two minutes
- Exercise 3: Burpees (two sets of ten reps each
- Exercise 4: Jump rope (three minutes)
- Rest for two minutes
- Exercise 5: Jumping jacks (two sets of ten reps each)
- Exercise 6: Burpees (three sets of eight reps each)

Day 5: Lower Body Workout

- Warm-up: Jumping jacks (five minutes)
- Exercise 1: Walking lunges (three sets of eight reps each)
- Exercise 2: Lunges (three sets of eight reps each)
- Rest for two minutes
- Exercise 3: Squats (three sets of eight reps each)
- Exercise 4: Bridges (three sets of eight reps each)

- Rest for two minutes
- Exercise 5: High knees (two sets of five reps each)
- Exercise 6: The donkey kick (three sets of five reps each)

Day 6: Upper body workout

- Warm-up: Jump rope (five minutes)
- Exercise 1: Side planks (three sets of ten reps each)
- Exercise 2: Superman (three sets of eight reps each)
- Rest for two minutes
- Exercise 3: Bird dog (two sets of eight reps each)
- Exercise 4: Bicycle crunch (two sets of ten reps each)
- Rest for two minutes
- Exercise 5: Jump rope (three minutes)
- Exercise 6: Wall pushups (three sets of eight reps each)

Day 7: Full body cardio workout

- Warm-up: Jump rope (five minutes)
- Exercise 1: Jumping jacks (three sets of ten reps each)
- Exercise 2: Burpees (three sets of ten reps each)
- Rest for two minutes
- Exercise 3: High knees (two sets of ten reps each)

- Exercise 4: Planks (hold for thirty seconds per rep, three reps)
- Rest for two minutes
- Exercise 5: Bicycle crunch (two sets of five reps each)
- Exercise 6: Bird dog (two sets of five reps each)

This exercise routine is meant for beginners, but everyone begins at different levels. Feel free to adjust the number of sets and reps to suit where you are in your exercise journey. After completing the first week, you can repeat the routine as is for week two or tweak the exercises. You know all you need to know to start your journey with intermittent fasting to achieve incredible results!

Leave a review!

Leave a 1-Click Review

Customer Reviews

★★★★★ 2
5.0 out of 5 stars ▾

5 star	100%
4 star	0%
3 star	0%
2 star	0%
1 star	0%

See all verified purchase reviews ›

Share your thoughts with other customers

Write a customer review

I would be incredibly thankful if you could take just 60 seconds to write a brief review on Amazon, even if it just a few sentences!

Scan the QR Code Below for a Quick Review!

Conclusion

Many diet books forget to accommodate the age factor and how age and a changing metabolism affect the body's response to an eating pattern. This book remedies that. Here, you have learned what intermittent fasting is and the different methods you can embrace to integrate this eating pattern into your life. We have discussed the changes you can expect in your body and shed light on how to deal with them from a dietary and fitness perspective. You have learned what food to eat and how you should plan out your meals. This book has even provided recipes that you can use so that all you have to do is shop for the ingredients and start living healthily.

Chapter six taught you how to slowly start switching to healthier habits. I have provided tips that you can use to make the transition smooth, easy, and seamless. The goal of this book is to empower you through knowledge. Now you understand why many diets do not work and why intermittent fasting works. You are now one of the many women who have the necessary tools to take more control of their health. Only one question remains: will you put that knowledge into practice? Will you commit to and trust the process until you become another intermittent fasting success story?

I hope that the answer is an emphatic yes. I hope you will be another candle lighting the health and fitness world with the good news that is IF. And I certainly hope that you loved this book enough to share it with women like you looking to understand IF. You can do that by leaving a review on Amazon. And I wish you all the best in your health journey!

Bibliography

(Ice), A. B. (n.d.). *Alternate-day fasting.* Healthline. https://www.healthline.com/nutrition/alternate-day-fasting-guide#health-benefits

(Ice), A. B. (n.d.). *The beginner's guide to the 5:2 diet.* Healthline. https://www.healthline.com/nutrition/the-5-2-diet-guide#TOC_TITLE_HDR_5

10 intermittent fasting benefits and potential risks. (2021, July 2). Healthy Meal Delivery - Trifecta Nutrition. https://www.trifectanutrition.com/blog/intermittent-fasting-benefits-and-potential-risks

5 myths about intermittent fasting debunked. (2021, September 28). femina.in. https://www.femina.in/wellness/diet/5-myths-about-intermittent-fasting-debunked-206766.html

5 stats that show why intermittent fasting is powerful for weight loss. (2019, July 23). Diet vs Disease. https://www.dietvsdisease.org/intermittent-fasting-is-powerful-for-weight-loss/

7 healthy habits for a healthy life. (2021, February 26). Living Magazine. https://www.livingmagazine.net/7-healthy-habits-healthy-life/

All the questions you have about intermittent fasting, answered. (2021, January 21). Catholic Health Today. https://blog.chsbuffalo.org/intermittent-fasting-faq/

Anonymous. (2016, November 16). *Lemon-herb rice salad.* Food Network. https://www.foodnetwork.com/recipes/food-network-kitchen/lemon-herb-rice-salad-recipe-2107971

Baier, L. (2021, October 21). *Intermittent fasting meal plan | How to create your eating routine | A sweet pea chef.* A Sweet Pea Chef. https://www.asweetpeachef.com/intermittent-fasting-meal-plan/

Bates, A., & CCN. (2020, May 29). *5 intermittent fasting break-fast recipes for EVERY situation! (Traveling, brunch, at work).* Autumn-ElleNutrition. https://www.autumnellenutrition.com/post/5-intermittent-fasting-break-fast-recipes-for-every-situation-traveling-brunch-at-work?ref=tfrecipes

Body changes after 50: How much can you control? (2021, December 8). Next Avenue. https://www.nextavenue.org/body-changes-50-control/

Brick, S. (n.d.). *Is alternate-day fasting really that good for you? We dig.* Greatist. https://greatist.com/health/alternate-day-fasting#what-is-adf

Does the 5:2 diet really help with weight loss? (2019, September 18). Verywell Fit. https://www.verywellfit.com/5-2-diet-pros-cons-and-how-it-works-4770014#toc-what-can-you-eat

Fasting facts: A few things you didn't know about intermittent fasting. (2019, April 24). Live Pure Low Down. https://livepure.love/blog/fasting-facts-a-few-things-you-didnt-know-about-intermittent-fasting/

Nazish, N. (2021). Forbes. https://www.forbes.com/sites/nomanazish/2021/06/30/10-intermittent-fasting-myths-you-should-stop-believing/?sh=22675c64335b

Gunnars, K. (2020). *Intermittent fasting 101 — The ultimate beginner's guide.* Healthline. https://www.healthline.com/nutrition/intermittent-fasting-guide#effects

Gunnars, K. (2021). *10 evidence-based health benefits of intermittent fasting.* Healthline. https://www.healthline.com/nutrition/10-health-benefits-of-intermittent-fasting#TOC_TITLE_HDR_10

Gunnars, K. (n.d.). *How intermittent fasting can help you lose weight.* Healthline. https://www.healthline.com/nutrition/intermittent-fasting-and-weight-loss#healthier-eating

How this woman used intermittent fasting to lose 80 pounds in a year. (2020, January 28). NBC News. https://www.nbcnews.com/better/lifestyle/how-one-woman-used-intermittent-fasting-lose-80-pounds-year-ncna1124121

Intermittent fasting 14/10: A step-by-step strategy to knock off those unwanted pounds. (2022, April 5). BetterMe Blog. https://betterme.world/articles/intermittent-fasting-14-10/

Intermittent fasting 14/10: All you need to know. (2022, May 3). 21 Day Hero. https://21dayhero.com/intermittent-fasting-14-10/

Intermittent fasting success stories. (n.d.). Diet Doctor. https://www.dietdoctor.com/intermittent-fasting/success-stories

Intermittent fasting: 4 different types explained. (2020, September 3). Cleveland Clinic. https://health.clevelandclinic.org/intermittent-fasting-4-different-types-explained/

Intermittent fasting: What is it, and how does it work? (n.d.). Johns Hopkins Medicine, based in Baltimore, Maryland. https://www.hopkinsmedicine.org/health/wellness-and-prevention/intermittent-fasting-what-is-it-and-how-does-it-work

JamieOliver.com. (2019, July 17). *Vegetarian pad Thai | Jamie Oliver vegetarian recipes.* Jamie Oliver. https://www.jamieoliver.com/recipes/vegetable-recipes/veggie-pad-thai/

Jennings, S., & The Courier-Journal. (2021, June 9). *'My health was off the rails and I knew it': How intermittent fasting changed everything.* Louisville Courier Journal. https://www.courier-journal.com/story/opinion/2021/06/09/intermittent-fasting-helped-me-lose-weight-improved-my-health/7596122002/

Kitchenatics. (2021, November 18). *Intermittent fasting weight loss second Part 16 over 8 method.* KITCHENATICS - Kitchen Products, Cookware, Baking Tools. https://kitchenatics.com/health-tips/16-8-method-intermittent-fasting/

Kubala, J. (2020). *9 potential intermittent fasting side effects.* Healthline. https://www.healthline.com/nutrition/intermittent-fasting-side-effects#Who-should-avoid-intermittent-fasting

Leonard, J. (n.d.). *16:8 intermittent fasting: Benefits, how-to, and tips.* Medical and health information. https://www.medicalnewstoday.com/articles/327398#diabetes

LibGuides: Fake news and alternative facts: Finding accurate news: Why is fake news harmful? (2021, 24). LibGuides at Austin Community College. https://researchguides.austincc.edu/c.php?g=612891&p=4258046

Link, R. (2021, January). *What are the different stages of intermittent fasting?* Healthline. https://www.healthline.com/nutrition/stages-of-fasting#The-bottom-line

Moody, L. (2019, August 27). *Bookmark this: The only formula you need for a perfect green smoothie, every time.* mindbodygreen. https://www.mindbodygreen.com/0-27424/bookmark-this-the-only-formula-you-need-for-a-perfect-green-smoothie-every-time.html

Need an intermittent fasting meal plan? Here's your 7-Day brunch and dinner plan to break your fast. (2020, January 30). Women's Health. https://www.womenshealthmag.com/weight-loss/a30658778/inter mittent-fasting-meal-plan-men-s-health/

Pannell, N. (2018, August 27). *10 things you've heard about intermittent fasting that aren't true.* Insider. https://www.insider.com/intermit tent-fasting-myths-2018-8#myth-intermittent-fasting-works-because-your-body-doesnt-process-foods-at-night-10

Park, W. (2019). *The benefits of intermittent fasting the right way.* https://www.bbc.com/future/article/20220110-the-benefits-of-intermittent-fasting-the-right-way

Snader, J. (2021). *The pros and cons of fasting.* Welcome to Forklift & Palate!. https://www.forkliftandpalate.com/manheim/blog/the-pros-and-cons-of-fasting

StreitN, L., & LD. (n.d.). *16/8 intermittent fasting: Meal plan, benefits, and more.* Healthline. https://www.healthline.com/nutrition/16-8-intermittent-fasting#recommendation

Ways you didn't know your body changes after 50. (2020, March 2). The Daily Meal. https://www.thedailymeal.com/healthy-eating/body-changes-after-50-gallery

What to expect in your 50s. (n.d.). WebMD. https://www.webmd.com/ healthy-aging/ss/slideshow-what-to-expect-in-your-50s

Why you should transition into intermittent fasting. (n.d.). Chiropractor | The Joint Chiropractic. https://www.thejoint.com/arizona/avon dale/gateway-crossing-48019/266212-why-you-should-transition-into-intermittent-fasting